LOVE AWAY UNWANTED FAT-
FOREVER !!

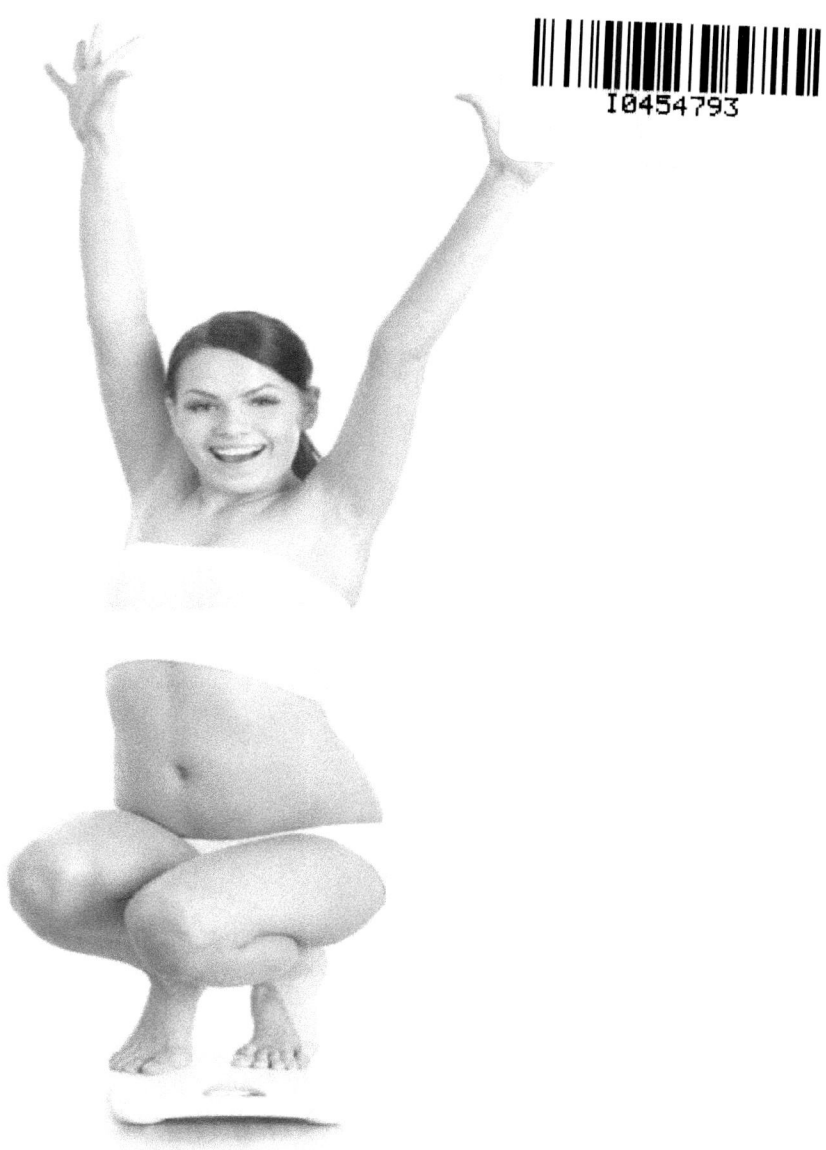

Published by
Joseph Gordon Prescott

Third Printing

Printed in U.S.A.

CONTENTS

FOREWORD

DIRECTIONS; HOW TO USE PART I

8.   INTRODUCTION/EXPLANATION

13.   THE ROOT CAUSE

17.   LOVE-O-ME-TER

22.   PIM-PREDOMENANT IMAGE MOTIVATOR

25.   WHY DO I OVER EAT?

31.   FOOD – SECURITY-LOVE

32.   YOUR SECURITY GUARD

34.   LOVE AWAY FAT PROGRAM

38.   COMPULSIVE EATING

39.   LOVE, ROMANCE, SEX

44.   THE PLUMP Teenager

45.   PART II, INNER MIND POWER AFFIRMATIONS

49.   LAF, LOVE is the CHANGING POWER

56.   LOVE IS THE LIBERATING POWER

59.   POSI-PEP, PUNISHMENT

64.   IDENTIFCATION

66.   YOU HAVE CONTROL

70.   YOU ACT ON YOUR LOVE

71.   LOVE IS GIVING

79.   MELT-AWAY-PROGRAM

82.   LOVE IS THE CHANGING POWER

83.   LOVE"ROMANCE SEX AFFIRMATIONS

90.   GOAL SETTING-MAP

91.   GOAL CARD 10

100.   MAKE MENTAL MOVIES

100.   LAF CARDS

131.   HURT MAP

136.   APPESTAT

137.   TOGETHERNESS EXERCISE

145.   NEGATE A NEGATIVE PROMPTER

146.   R. AND R. SESSONS

147.   YOUR HEART'S DESIRE

FOREWORD

Joe Prescott, in LAUFF (Love Away Unwanted Fat Forever) tackles the hopeless feeling most overweight folks have when they dare look at their situation.
Prescott zeroes in on the root cause, a lack of love, or misapplied love. He provides a roadmap out of this dark forest. In addition to love that is lacking or misapplied, in this book which is really a workbook, we meet the powerful pair—the PEP and the PIM. We are all aware of the power of emotions, and Dr. Prescott helps us face both healthy and unhealthy predominant emotional prompters, the PEPs. He also helps us get in touch with our Predominant Image
Motivators, the PIMs.

A powerful truth saturates these pages: when logic and emotions clash, the emotions win out! And when our will power and imagination clash, the imagination wins out! The LAF-BOOK and the HURT MAP help folks work on our emotional framework.

The re-writing of our life scripts and the establishing of an atmosphere of positive affirmation make up the second part of the book, and of the program. From the over-weight teenager to the marriage in trouble, there is hope and help in the program Prescott outlines. Script cards, LAF cards, and Love cards help folks get serious about emotional and physical health, and begin to change their life with God's help.

Earl C. Davis, B.A., B.D., PhD.

Acknowledgments

The author gratefully acknowledges the contributions of the following individuals who willingly offered suggestions and reviewed the material:

I see that you have again qualified for certification in both the Association to Advance Ethical Hypnosis and the International Society for Professional Hypnosis. Requirements for certification each year keeps you abreast of information that is quite valuable to you and your clients.

George W. Knox, Ph.D. Psychologist

Thousands are benefiting from this method, including myself.
Garland H. Fross, D.D.S., Past President,
Fellow and Faculty member, A.I.H.

"As a Licensed Clinical Social Worker (LCSW) and a Certified Hypnotherapist, I recommend The Love Away Unwanted Fat Forever book due to its unique qualities in meeting the important needs of the emotional, behavioral and spiritual aspects of losing weight. It most importantly addresses the spiritual needs of the participant which is paramount in lasting change. If you are seeking lasting change, this book is easy to read and gives good examples of how to implement in one's daily life."
Charlotte Bailey, LCSW
Clinical Hypnotherapis

Finally, a book that addresses the root of our nation's obesity problem! Using his years of experience as a hypnotherapist and church-setting marriage and family therapist, Dr. Prescott addresses ones feelings of "not being loved" as the root cause and how to overcome these feelings!

Though designed specifically for those struggling to overcome unwanted weight, the principles are applicable to ALL of us. Most of us have past hurts that were never properly healed. With Prescott's guidance we can begin this healing process and begin to forgive ourselves and/or others for the events of the past. With Prescott's plan, you will: Stop trying - Stop dieting and

Love Away Unwanted Fat FOREVER!!

Mary Catherine   Gatlin, Ed.D.

LAUFF- the light at the end of the obesity epidemic.
Dr. Joe Prescott in his book LAUFF (Love Away Unwanted Fat Forever) looks at the truth behind why so many of us overindulge- the lack of self-appreciation and love. By usingthis book as a guide and workbook, I believe the readers will not only find themselves losing weight but also being happier in all aspects of life!

Laura B. Youngblood, MD

EXCERPTS FROM LETTERS OF CLIENTS:

"I am now at my goal weight and have stayed there.   I've changed my three worst habits of eating.   The thing that is

6

so thrilling for me is that I really feel that I will never again be overweight.   This makes me feel better as a total person."

C. D.

"I can't tell you how wonderful I feel.   Dr. Prescott, you have changed my whole outlook on life.   Before,   I   was too fat and exhausted to go any place after a day's work.   I just stayed home, ate, and watched T.V. I love the new person I'm becoming. It is so wonderful to know that I now have complete control of my eating habits."

M. H.

"I would like this card to express the peace that you have helped foster in my mind during our association."

Pat

FROM THE OLD MASTERS:

"Human beings can alter their lives by altering their attitudes of mind."
William James

"When a man starts and continues a self-improvement program, his future is unlimited."

Benjamin Franklin

HOW TO USE LAUFF BOOK

The purpose of PART I is to give you a good foundation for the POSITIVE AFFIRMATIONS in PART II. Read PART I at least once all the way through before starting to read PART II.. Thus you will get a better understanding of the principles involved - and why the LOVE AWAY FAT M.A.P. (My Achievement Program) is successful, while so many of the reducing and diet plans fail miserably.

Read and devote thought to it when you can do so while concentrating without effort and without undue distractions. You want to get the message clearly into your inner mind. After reading in this manner at least once, you may benefit by reading certain parts for emphasis.

The instructions on pages 132 to 138 can help you make the material much more effective.
So READ and LOVE AWAY FAT!

LOVE AWAY UNWANTED FAT FOREVER

!!!

INTRODUCTION/EXPLANATION

You probably have found by now that dieting and exercise, alone OR together, are not the answer to your overweight concern. But now you can have HOPE, real ASSURANCE, knowing that you have the right way to cope with your concerns.

Dieting and exercise, along with the many, many other methods, or variations of these in thousands of programs on TV, in magazines, books and newspapers DO NOT correct and eliminate the ROOT CAUSE, the basic cause of overeating and/or overweight. In fact, according to medical doctors who have researched this area, some of these methods cause illnesses!

"Well", you might say, "Isn't overeating the cause? Why do you mention both overeating and overweight? Aren't they the same?" Not necessarily! Overeating itself may be a symptom of a deeper underlying cause. Some people really have the problem of overeating, while others have the problem of overweight. The overeating will cause the overweight, but in their case, overeating is the concern to be dealt with.

Regardless of which concern is yours, LOVE AWAY FAT succeeds. The overweight person almost for certain will

come to feel it is HOPELESS after *trying* and *trying* over and over again. In fact the word "try" indicates the very possibility of failure! So the first thing you will learn with "Loving Away Fat" is to get rid of the negative "try."

Pause for a moment, and think of the many things you do well, things you do automatically without conscious effort, WITHOUT "trying." You don't TRY to dress yourself; you DRESS yourself. You do so automatically, not even "trying" or consciously thinking about which sleeve goes on first, or which pants leg goes on first. Yet it is the same every time, isn't it? The same applies to driving the car, brushing your teeth, and thousands of other things!

Millions of dollars are spent every year by people "trying' to "lose weight." The Love Away Fat M.A.P. is a means to stop spending, stop "trying" and having <u>a way of maintaining your ideal size and weight</u>. Forget the word DIET. It is another negative and counterproductive word. Take the "T" off the word diet, and see what you have. No one wants that! Furthermore, who really wants to diet anyway? Call it "nutriment," "nutrition-support "regime, or "regimen." I like the regimen definition: "the characteristic behavior or orderly procedure of a natural phenomenon or process". Call it 'The M.A.P. way", but leave diet out of your vocabulary!

Eugene Scheimann, M.D., puts it this way: "Dieting is not the answer to a weight problem because <u>dieting is not a way of life</u>. It is rather a desperate, stopgap measure which is doomed to failure; We must find a way of eating that we can <u>live</u> with, day after day, year after year. We must find a way of enjoying food without destroying our peace of mind." 1

With the "LOVE AWAY FAT" MAP or regimen, you can now have HOPE, and more importantly, rather than being on a seesaw of ups and downs with your weight, you can look forward to PERMANENT success!

"I get angry with myself"

Maybe you or an overweight loved one has reached such a state of hopelessness that the DESIRE is lacking. Rationalization has taken over: "I feel OK with the extra weight." "He loves me the way I am." "What's the use?" Continue on along with LAF. You are in for a pleasant surprise! Even if one is not overweight, the LAF MAP can be of tremendous benefit in other areas of life. You are going to find HELP for yourself, and you can recommend LAF to friends with other habit concerns.

Going through my files and recordings of sessions of overweight people who have come to me with this concern, I find many evidences of their <u>not loving themselves properly</u>. It shows up in statements like the following:

> "I get angry with myself"
>
> "I'm always a disappointment." "It's almost like a self-destruct." "I'm not a disciplined person."
>
> "I want to stop punishing myself" "I dislike myself;

I feel guilty."
"I don't feel like a person, I feel like a nobody."
"I'm disgusted with myself"
"I hate myself"

Especially after holidays, or a "lost weekend" there are bouts of self-recrimination. There are many "I should not haves", and the self-flagellating continues.

Here are a couple of quotes of folks who really *TRYING*:
"1 want to like myself better."
"I want to feel loved."
Note she did not say that she was not LOVED; she didn't FEEL LOVED. How we FEEL is more important than plain reason-logic, what the facts really are.
Then there are those who get the principle "Love people and use things" backwards, and use people or at least, love things. They say:
"I love chocolate." "I love sweets."
"I love food!"
"Ice cream, I love it"

Notice the "it". Subconsciously honest, this person "loves" sex, but under hypnosis revealed that he was not participating in the triune of LOVE, ROMANCE and SEX. As a consequence, there was an unfilled lack, a "hunger" that longed to be satisfied. This Predominant Emotional Prompter (PEP) prompted him to *TRY* (note try) to fulfill that lack by orally consuming the tastiest thing available. His "trying" did not work. He just got bigger, and he was still not satisfied!

Dr. Leo Buscaglia, in his book, "LOVE" says, "So most of us never learn to love at all. Is it any wonder so many of us are dying of loneliness, feel anxious and UNFULFILLED, even in seemingly close relationships, and are <u>always looking</u>

elsewhere for something more which we feel must certainly be there? 'Is that all there is?' the song asks," (Note the words "UNFULFILLED" and "Always looking elsewhere for something." These words echo what many of my clients FEEL and DO.)

DR. Buscaglia continues, "LOVE offers itself as a continual feast to be nourished upon. ".2

THE ROOT CAUSE

While everyone is different, and different "reasons" are given for being overweight, still there is the one deep real ROOT CAUSE, A LACK OF LOVE or MISAPPLIED LOVE. This does not mean that you do not love, love God, and love others. Even ministers have discovered with this LAF-MAP that unconsciously they were misapplying love.

This may take on many forms, or other names may be used to describe it: *insecurity, frustration, boredom, rejection, resentment, hostility, loneliness, anxiety, depression, sexual problems.* Any one or more of these may cause overeating and/or wrong eating patterns. These in turn cause more of the same, creating a vicious cycle.

Richard Murkiness, in "Eat Fat and Grow Slim", says "The biggest single reason for overeating is a feeling of love dieting, and if your subconscious has accepted the 'fact' that ' food is love', then you can see why <u>dieting does not work</u>."

"We are shaped and fashioned by what we love", states Johann Wolfgang Von Oaethe.[2]

Many feel unwanted and rejected. As one man put it, "You only have one childhood, and when someone messes that up----." Here a person is still carrying deep resentment and bitterness in his forties, and finding it awfully hard to get rid of those negative feelings caused by being hurt. He is **unwilling to forgive and let go**, unable now to love and receive love in a proper way, yet he is starved for love.
It may be that you were hurt in another way. A lady who never could have children of her own, due to an operation while in her teens, now at forty-nine, although happily married and with adopted children, is still *trying* to fulfill a lack in her life -with food and being "pregnantly fat"!

A man states, "I feel I am selfish to ask God to help me. Wife has wrong background, hang-ups on sex. It's bigger than I am. I like sex, food, happiness at home. So I snack." "When." I asked. (I could have told him when, but I wanted him to get it out.) "Mostly at night, usually when by myself; wife goes to bed, and I'm sitting there watching TV—". You could probably finish that statement for him: "hungry, unfilled, wanting love and affection, romance and sex." "Food is love", so he thinks and fills his mouth with food—sweets, rather than kisses!

In the book "LOVE or PERISH", by Smiley Blanton, M.D., Dr. Blanton states, "Love, in our psychic life, is the great combining force that seeks to join all parts together. It is the organizing element in our emotional structure. It is the power that reaches out to build and construct. Love is the immortal flow of energy that <u>nourishes, extends. and preserves.</u> It's eternal goal is life."[3]

You have been hurt some way, somehow, sometime. Before you go further in this LAF-MAP, before you read further, sit down with your LAF ACHIEVEMENT-BOOK and in private, start writing. Also refer to "Hurt Map" in back of the book. Write about how you have been hurt. What was the situation? Who was involved? What situation offended you, anything unworthy as cruelty or meanness? It doesn't matter whether it was intentional or unintentional, real or assumed. Maybe it was an injustice, an injury or disappointment, some frustration or "sin". Ready? Stop and write, take your time. Let it all out. Then, only then, resume reading LAF BOOK.
By the way, we recommend very strongly that you show your list to no one. It is just between you and God! OK, start writing.

Have you done the exercise? If you have, you should feel better already; at least you will as time goes on. It will have a relief-valve effect. If you did not write it down and said something like, "Oh, I know, it's in my head", stop, DO IT. WRITE. There is something therapeutic about writing it down.

Now, you are ready for the next close look.
What were your FEELINGS at that time, or over the time span affected?   Did you feel rejected?
Hurt? Angry? Disappointed? Resentful?

Stop again and take time NOW to write down your exact FEELINGS. Use as many words as you can think of to describe the feelings that you had <u>at that time</u>, and since. OK, stop now.
Be honest with yourself, and write them down.

IF you feel that you just must tell someone, confess them to a minister, a priest, a rabbi or a counselor who you know will keep confidences, someone other than friend or family. This is important. Some of the negative feelings may have vanished from your conscious memory. Others you may still remember.
To help bring forgotten information back into your conscious memory, use the "Togetherness Exercise" found later in LAF-BOOK. As you relax physically and mentally, your memory works better. As the situations and feelings come to mind, write them down.

Did you find that a "hurt" that came to your mind was some wrong that you have done in your own life, against yourself only, or against someone else also?
How many of these feelings do you still have, consciously or subconsciously? Are you still chafing? Blaming? Condemning? Or punishing *you*?

15

The very act of carrying out the preceding exercise can have a tremendous cleansing effect. For many, this is all that is needed to cause a turnabout in behavior. For reinforcement and for handling the Negative-Predominant Emotional Prompters and Negative-Predominant Image Motivators in your life, the positive affirmations elsewhere help you to LOVE YOURSELF MORE and **LOVE AWAY FAT!**

Check yourself on some other negative emotions, some of which are merely variations of the foregoing: worry, anxiety, apprehension, discouragement, disappointment, frustration, loneliness, shame, and especially guilt; being hurt, upset, disillusioned, downcast, gloomy, disgusted.
Also check remorse, bitterness, hostility. or rejection,
See the "My LOVE-O-ME-TER". Are you using food to *TRY* to escape, to bring comfort and solace or as a sedative?

MY LOVE O-ME-TER

CHECK OR CIRCLE NUMBER INDICATING HOW YOU FEEL.

1-SOMETIMES   2-OCCASIONALLY   3-MOST OF TIME

HURT	—3—2—1	0+1+2+3	LOVED
CONFUSED	—3—2—1	0+1+2±3	UNDERSTOOD
DISAPPOINTED	—3—2—1	01+2+3	SATISFIED
INDIGNANT	—3—2—1	0+1+2+3	PURPOSEFUL
EMBARRASSED	—3—2—1	0~1+2+3	CONFIDENT
UPSET	-3—2---1	0+1+2+3	PLEASED
REJECTED	—3—2—1	0+1+2~3	ACCEP TED
DOWNCAST	—3—2—1	0+1+2+3	HAPPY
ANXIOUS	—3—2—1	0+1+2+3	DETERMINED
ANGRY	—3—2—1	0+1+2+3	CALM
FURIOUS	—3—2—1	0+1+2+3	SERENE
RAGING	—3—2—1	0+1+2+3	TRANDUIL
FRUSTRATED	—3—2—1	0+1+2+3	COLLECTED
RESENTFUL	—3—2—1	0+1+2+3	CORDIAL
SELF-HATING	—3—2—1	0+1+2+3	SELF—LOVING
VENGEFUL	—3—2—1	0+1+2+3	HELPFUL
BITTER	—3—2—1	0+1+2+3	FORGIVING
JEALOUS	—3—2—1	0+1+2+3	TRUSTING
SPITEFUL	—3—2—1	0+1÷2~3	CARING
ENVIOUS	—3—2—1	0+1~2~3	GIVING
SELFISH	—3—2—1	0+1+2+3	SHARING
INDIFFERENT	—3—2—1	0+1+2+3	CONCERNED

"Against these hostile emotions neither laws nor logic can prevail", says Dr. Smiley Blanton, psychiatrist for over forty-nine years. He follows with, "Once in the grip of hostility, we twist forward in a spiral of destructive action. Nothing can stop the spiral except love."[4]

These negative feelings, these emotional hang-ups, in whatever way they show themselves, -fear, resentment, bitterness, any lack of love or misapplied love, have become your NEGATIVE PREDOMINANT EMOTIONAL **PROMPTERS,** abbreviated as NEGA-PEP.

The **EMOTIONS PROMPT** our **BEHAVIOR.**

When there is a conflict in one's life, the **PREDOMINANT EMOTIONAL Prompters** overrule and win! They overcome LOGIC, REASON, and COMMON SENSE. We develop habits of these thoughts and feelings, which result in INNER ATTITUDES. Our INNER ATTITUDES affect our BEHAVIOR.

To overcome a bad habit or rid yourself of a mental block, to improve in a certain area of your life, you simply replace the NEGA-PEPS with POSI-PEPS, or make the POSI-PEPS stronger than the NEGA-PEPS. Note that I said "simply", and it will also be easy, as you build love and confidence following this Love Away Fat MAP.

Napoleon Hill, in "Think and Grow Rich", lists these as the seven major negative emotions: fear, jealousy, hatred, revenge, greed, superstition, angers. There is no love found here!

Nathaniel Brandon in "The Psychology of Self-Esteem" states, "The single most formidable obstacle to identifying the roots of one's emotions is repression".[6]

Please don't let the ugly monster of repression or rationalization come between you and the discovering of your PEP.

18

In "Faith Is The Answer", Norman Vincent Peale and Smiley Blanton state, "It is not easy to be absolutely honest with ourselves, due to the process of rationalization".[7]

NOW is the time to FACE, not FLEE, nor FIGHT, nor *TRY* to FORGET, but **FACE** realistically, honestly, the Predominant Emotional Prompters and the Predominant Image Motivators in your life, and make that change, loving away fat! Analogous to repentance, a conversion, it is a turning around and away from the defeating negative emotions and images and their consequences, and turning toward the greatest Positive Emotional Prompter of all -LOVE.

THE EMOTIONS ARE THE MOST POWERFUL, MOVING FORCES WITHIN US, AND LOVE IS THE GREATEST EMOTION. THUS LOVE IS THE GREATEST MOVING FORCE!

Dr. James Mallory, psychiatrist, in "The Kink and I", says, "Love is the most powerful healing force that exists in an individual's life."
"The greatest of these is love."[9]

What are the rewards and benefits to be derived? Ask yourself: "What's in it for my family, my loved ones, for me?!" Stop again and write these down. Some of these are antonyms to the negatives written before. Saturate these POSI-PEPS with love. "Perfect love casts out fear." To LOVE also casts out the many other negative emotions that mutilate or cripple.

No one is perfect, and you can be thankful that you are "as perfect" as you are. Since no one is perfect, why condemn yourself by such attitudes as "I'm angry at myself, I dislike Myself, etc., etc."

Dr. Wayne Dyer. author of "Your Erroneous Zones" says," You have to really like yourself a lot and be in charge of yourself, and **not** let other people run your life." So LOVE is the answer, the key. He further states, "Take a look at all the emotional reactions that you have in your life: those which you don't like, those which are immobilizing, and those which don't work. Stop defending them." [11]

By reading the LAF affirmations regularly, you rid yourself of self-defeating behavior.
You are ridding yourself of useless or "immobilizing" actions!
Refer to "Hurt Map" again. Read directions and peruse the map and reference signs.

PIM,
PREDOMINANT IMAGE MOTIVATOR

The other powerful force in your inner mind that we want to deal with is the Predominant Image Motivator- PIM. It is the twin to PEP, more like Siamese twins, each one affects the other. When one is negative, you can be sure the other is also negative. Both are affected by our memory, conscious or subconscious memory of past experiences. We remember the hurts, the traumatic experiences, the embarrassing experiences. For example, we may respond to hostility with a hostility of our own. We may react to being upset and hurt with anger and revenge. We play the game of "getting even". Guilt comes into our lives, and we don't like what we see or feel in ourselves. We then develop a MENTAL IMAGE of ourselves which is the sum total of images over the years. We act according to this mental image, this script, this identity we have of ourselves.

We have different images of ourselves in different situations. Some are more powerful than others, and we call these Predominant Image Motivators or PIMS.

For example, one may see himself as a non-drinker, and have no trouble passing by a bar; and at the same time see himself as a smoker and automatically take a cigarette when offered his brand. One may see himself as a non-smoker and also see himself as one who "loves Cokes", and can hardly pass a vending machine without getting a Coke!

The PEP and PIM work together, stirring you over-whelmingly to feel a certain *way,* and perceive yourself as acting out your script in specific situations, so as to fulfill that PROMPTER and that MOTIVATOR.

Remember, when there is a conflict between logic and emotions, *the emotions win out!*

When there is a conflict between will power and the imagination *the imagination wins out!*

When there is a conflict between the conscious mind and the subconscious mind, the subconscious overrules the conscious *trying*! The PEP and PIM are overpowering! Therefore, you see the tremendous need to make sure we have the right PEPS and PIMS operating within.

See "HOW TO CREATE and SECURE IN YOUR MIND a desired POSITIVE PROMPTER/MOTIVATOR".

Let's look at another aspect of your PEP. The NEGA-PEPS may not really be negative in and of themselves. Nor were they negative in the past; but when they hinder you from being your better self NOW, we consider them NEG-A-PEPS. They must be overpowered with a POSITIVE EMOTIONAL PROMPTER.

Napoleon Hill lists these as---POSITIVE EMOTIONS:
desire, enthusiasm, faith, hope, love, sex, and romance."

I am quoting many sources of truth proven by years of experience and including quotes from the Bible. Whether you believe the Bible or not, these truths still work. They will work for you even if you are a non-believer in God.

23

I do, however, wish that you may have the same assurance, peace, security, and joy that I have. By turning from MY WAY and turning to God through Jesus Christ, By just trusting in Him and giving Him control of my life, as best I can and with His help is a positive PEP/PIM..

E. Stanley Jones, in his book, "Victory Through Surrender", puts it this way: "The sense of not belonging to anything real and eternal is the central insecurity of our time. The first need is to belong. Belong to what? If your surrender is to anything this side of God, it will let you down.

No matter how good the thing to which you attach your ultimate loyalty is, if it is this side of God, it will let you down.   Self-surrender is the central necessity in life."

Paraphrased: "Surrender to LOVE, to Jesus Christ who is LOVE, and not to your appetites and impulses. When you belong to Christ everything belongs to you."[13] "He who does not love does not know God; for God is love. In this the love of God was made manifest among us, that God sent his only son into the world, so that we might live through him. In this is love, not that we loved God but that he loved us and sent his son to be the expiation for our sins." [14]

Many of my clients say such things as, "I'm disgusted with myself", "I hate myself for-doing it", and the many other condemnations of self. Loving yourself more, you realize you should have compassion for the child-self within you.

You know the ad that goes, "I could have had a__" As a loving adult, and with the LAF MAP, you keep yourself from getting in that position.

You don't have to look back and say, "I could have had the joy and happiness of a loving adult.

WHY DO I OVER-EAT?

Some people are still striving for the joy and happiness they had, or thought they had, as a child. Others are looking for that Joy and happiness they might not have had, but yearned for as children. "We know that the most powerful influence on our actions and behavior in life is the power of love; that everything we do in life is either to get love or to compensate for a lack of love"[15]

With the LAF MAP and LOVING YOURSELF MORE,
you NOW can have that Joy and happiness!

STOP READING AT THIS PONT, and go to "APPLIED LAF-TER, POINTS TO PONDER"
Then complete THINK ABOUT THESE THINGS, GAINING INSIGHT," and "THINGS TO DO".

APPLIED LAF-TER. <u>POINTS TO PONDER: WHAT HAVE I LEARNED</u>?
    1. MY WEIGHT CONCERN is NOT that my WILL POWER is weak or inoperative, I have been letting my FEELINGS and my MENTAL IMAGERY control ME.
I can control these with LOVING AWAY FAT, thus I have a way to control my weight from now on.

    2. Getting and maintaining my IDEAL WEIGHT is NOT_a matter of WILL or TRYING or DIETING. It is replacing the NEGATIVE INNER FEELING, that Negative Predominant Emotional Prompter with the greatest emotion of all, and the greatest PROMPTER of all, LOVE.

3.   The word *"TRY"* is negative, indicating possibility of FAILURE. "Trying" to "lose weight" is a negative, counter success phrase, so with LOVE AWAY FAT, I develop a positive successful way for life!

4.   I'm FREE to LOVE myself more and free to LET GO of wrong eating patterns.

5.   So in surrendering to LOVE, and creating in my mind a clear MENTAL IMAGE of my GOAL-IMAGE, I AM REWRITING MY SCRIPT, AND LOVING MYSELF   MORE and LOVING AWAY FAT!

APPLIED   LAF-TER: <u>THINK   ABOUT   THESE   THINGS;   GAINING   INSIGHT</u>:

Please circle a number from one (1) to seven (7) to indicate the degree that you experience these things. One (1) means "little" and seven (7) means a "Lot".

LITTLE---LOT
I.   Do I carry strong feelings about being hurt?
1234567
2.   How much do I still think about the situation?
1 2 3 4 5 6 7
3.   Do I still feel negative toward those involved?
1234567
4, Am   I   letting   a   NEGATIVE   PREDOMINANT   EMOTIONAL PROMPTER control me?
1234567
5. Do I find myself telling others about it VERY OFTEN?
1234567

6. The extent that I still feel rejected?
   1234567
7. The extent that I still feel angry?
   1234567
S. The extent that I still feel disappointed?
   1234567
9. The extent that I still feel resentful?
   1234567
10. The extent that I still feel guilty?
    1234567

THINGS TO DO:
Face the real PREDOMINANT EMOTIONAL PROMPTERS and
PREDOMINANT IMAGE MOTIVATORS.

Step 1. Using LAF-BOOK, and HURT MAP, put in your LAF ACHIEVEMENT BOOK, HOW YOU HAVE BEEN HURT.
Who offended? WHAT? Anything unworthy as cruelty or meanness; intentional or unintentional: real or assumed. Was it a disappointment, frustration, sin? WRITE it down secretly.

Step 2. Talk about these things with a minister, a priest, a rabbi or other counselor ANGER, GUILT, SELF-PUNISH-MENT

Step 3. Become keenly aware of any blaming or condemning of others! ONLY COMPLIMENT OTHERS!

Step 4. Actively ask yourself the question, "Am I punishing myself by this activity?"

Step 5. Read and REPEAT DAILY your GOAL CARD AFFIRMATION, Goal Card 10.
27

Have your favorite LAF CARDS and SCRIPT CARDS with you at all times, using them as indicated..

Turn the negative Predominant Emotional Prompters and the negative Predominant Image Motivators into POSITIVES with LOVE.

LOVING MYSELF MORE, I achieve the above by practicing the routine exercises in LAF BOOK, and using the "TRIGGER" procedure as outlined.
So I'll surrender to LOVE, not to my appetite and negative impulses.

THINGS TO TALK ABOUT:
What were my FEELINGS at THAT TIME and over the time affected?
Did I feel REJECTED, HURT, DISAPPOINTED, RESENTFUL ANGRY, and/or GUILTY?
How many of these feelings do I still have?
Especially look For ANGER and GUILT.
Anger against parents, even after the person is well up in years, is one of the most common causes of guilt. And guilt calls for punishment!- or *forgiveness!* It is amazing how many people seem to over-look this aspect of love. Forgive. Forgive. For heaven's sake, forgive! Forgive parents. Forgive self for having anger toward parents.

FORGIVE: FULLY, FREELY and FINALLY

A negative Predominant Emotional Prompter may be self-punishment for guilt one has for one of the other Predominant Emotional Prompters, such as the mutilation of one's body. From earliest times, as evidenced in primitive tribes in the cutting of their faces, lips and bodies, it indicates a way of punishment for wrongs not righted, or deeds which one *feels* are sins to rid themselves of GUILT!

It still goes on, perhaps in an updated, socially acceptable manner. Dr. Fray Alexander, a well-known leader in the field of psychosomatic medicine, states that mutilation is brought about "by a sense of guilt which the victim tries to expiate by self-imposed punishment".

We learn while growing up from actions of our parents. Child does something wrong, knows he is guilty, and feels *separated from love of parent*. Parent punishes child, Child is made to suffer to become "good", and thus regains love of parent. This is not necessarily the way it really is, but the way the child perceives it. The child has to have care and LOVE to survive psychologically as well as physically. In certain situations all the attention (or LOVE) he gets is when punished! That is enough to make one angry! This anger toward his parents creates more guilt, and so a vicious circle is created. Since guilt also calls for punishment, and he desires punishment, the acceptance of punishment becomes a way of *security* and survival, a way of obtaining LOVE. It is a way to <u>feel loved</u> and cared for. These are powerfully strong inner- mind prompters or motivators. Anger and guilt are spiritual and emotional "twins". Buried deeply within, they remain on into adult life.

Anger divides, defeats, destroys!

The negative Predominant Emotional Prompter says, "Getting food is being cared for, feeling *secure* and *loved;* so get food!" The subconscious mind says, "You've been injured, harmed, wronged; your feelings are wounded, you hurt, *food salves, soothes, slakes, satisfies, allays, assuages."* At the same time the twins, anger and guilt, cause an intense desire for self-punishment. Since food does not calm or pacify, *this* expresses itself by eating <u>more and more</u> and mutilating the body by becoming obese.

This heaps even more guilt on, as expressed by the saying, "I eat and I feel guilty."

BREAK THE VICIOUS CYCLE!!

Love gives. Love cares. **LOVE FORGIVES**. However the inner mind, perceiving love in a twisted and adulterated way, misuses love. Now is the time to put love in its proper perspective. The marriage of Anger and Guilt produces the children, Resentment and Bitterness. These in turn produce the children of Hostility, Rejection, Rebellion, and Revenge. (See additional quotes on this subject matter, and "HURT MAP", with "Road Signs" References).

The Bible tells us to "put them ALL away from you: anger, wrath, malice, slander." [i]
"Never avenge yourselves, but leave it to the wrath of God." [2]

Dr. Polston, in "There Can Be a New You" says, "The more you blame others, the greater the possibility grows for self-hate. Blaming people causes more mistakes which cause more blame" [3-] another vicious circle!

Beware of the parent-self who demands perfection. You realize this is a millstone to loving and accepting yourself more. It is a way of self-punishment. Face this question: Have you built into yourself a self-destruct system, demanding perfection whereby guaranteeing automatic failure, self-punishment? When you go by the "mental trash dump" and dump your anger, guilt and fear, and then go load up with "Forgiveness", you have also gotten rid of emotional tension. Furthermore, "...If you forgive men their trespasses, your- heavenly Father also will forgive you ".[4] That's a good deal!

Now you can see how overeating and/or overweight can be a subconscious way of trying to cope with the "child-self. The child-self FEELS the need for punishment for the anger and guilt, because he has the *feeling* that these thoughts are being bad and unacceptable, thus bringing separateness. The subconscious says, "Punishment will bring acceptance, togetherness and love; it did in the past." Go to your LAF ACHIEVMENT BOOK, where you have written down your feelings, and check for feelings of anger, guilt and other negatives that are similar.

FOOD-SECURITY-LOVE

It is not correct to regard overweight as if it were a problem of nutrition only. There is an abundance of evidence that diets alone do not work. It is a problem of LACK OF LOVE or the misuse of love. This takes on many forms, many names, but the root cause is the same. That is why so many, many programs that are on the market fail. Dieting and counting calories alone are counter to success. They tear at the heart of the concern- LOVING SELF PROPERLY.

I am not saying that if you are overweight, you don't love, or that you don't love yourself. Nor do I say that the lean person loves, and the fat person does not. No, but the fact remains that most of us, if not all, DO NOT LOVE AS **WE** SHOULD!

We are created in love, by love, for love, to love. We are created in the "Image of God"[1], and God is LOVE! [2] He tells us to love -- to love Him,[3] and why shouldn't we? Look what He has done for us. The Bible says, He made us a little less than Himself [4], and superior to everything else in the world! God tells us to LOVE others, and why shouldn't we? We get it back multiplied.[6] We are also to LOVE ourselves,.[7] .and why shouldn't we? We can complete the cycle and reap all the benefits.

With the LOVE AWAY FAT MAP, you have a way-of-life, not just a temporary program, a diet, or - technique or exercise. You have a WAY OF LIFE

ALL of us need and want LOVE, although we may not believe **it** or act like **it,** or receive love when it is presented. We must have LOVE — or cease to really live, or deteriorate, or go around as living zombies, or die untimely. When we are *separated* from love, we are miserable. Many people are going in many directions TRYING to over-come separation and lack of love, some seemingly going in many directions at the same time! The love in us may be handled properly, or it may be perverted, misused or misguided, but it must be dealt with. It will be dealt with; the question is HOW.

Jesus laid it before us: LOVE, LOVE, LOVE!
SO LOVE IS **THE CHANGING POWER:**
> LOVE of God ~ftom God, to God.
> LOVE of others —to others, from others.
> LOVE of self — to self, from self, ALL of yourself, the adult self and the child-self.
> What is that powerful force that drives you to eat when it is NOT for nutrition? The extreme is FEAR, fear of death, physical or spiritual -survival, the opposite of LOVE. There are many degrees, ranging from mild apprehension to deep anxieties.

Theodore J. Smith, M.D., says. "Spiritual LOVE is more powerful than physical LIFE. It is the most powerful force on the face of the earth!" We learn the habit from birth that to take food is to have LOVE: eat to love, to return love. "Food is the money of love, the medium of exchange, the currency of caring, whether it is given or received." states Dr. Smith.

Therefore when anything interferes with love- spiritual existence, food as love is taken in to fulfill (fill full) that lack. If hurt, whether it is anger, embarrassment, resentment, hostility, guilt or other spiritual negative subtracting from one's life, ANYTHING opposite the *security of Love*, the inner mind and subconscious memory reminds the person that "food is love, get food!". The subconscious says, "Food is comfort, get food"; "food is affection, get food"; "food is *security, get food!*"

Think of all the ways you learned about the many forms in which LOVE has been manifested in your life, comfort, caring, calming, sympathy. Now that you are older, no longer a small dependent child, you realize that food is for nutrition only. Your adult-self puts away from your child-self the subconscious thoughts of relating food to love. Your child-self *feels cared for, comforted, sympathized with, secure and loved,* knowing that all needs are taken care of by God through your adult-self. You feel pleased, happy, safe and secure. You feel LOVED!

Even when your adult-self feels neglected in the triune of LOVE, ROMANCE and SEX, you are firm with your child-self and block any attempts of making food a substitute. **_FOOD is NOT LOVE_**. Food is not ROMANCE. Food is not SEX. Food is food and too much or the wrong kind for you causes concerns-- bringing less self-esteem, less LOVE of SELF, feeling unlovely and /or unlovable, therefore,

YOU LOVE YOURSELF NOW.
YOU FEEL LOVED !

YOUR SECURITY GUARD

When you visit a big building where a large corporation is housed, you may find you have to register and get clearance through a security guard. Just as a security guard accepts "acceptable people" (those who can show proper credentials) and directs them to the proper place, the "security guard" of your mind allows "acceptable thoughts" to enter into your INNER-SELF. The problem with many people, however, is that they have been and are very careless about keeping a "security guard" on duty at all times. Therefore many unacceptable, negative thoughts just slip right on in, and many "O.K." thoughts are lost, since they are not properly directed into the INNER-MIND- the subconscious.

Carrying the analogy a little further, many large corporations, banks, etc. have their own internal security system. Yet occasionally you read that some disloyal person "on the inside" embezzled a large sum of money, or sold, or even gave away valuable secrets. In the same way many times we have negative thoughts of fear, doubt and other negative emotions, which rob us of large amounts of courage, perseverance, self-discipline, and self-confidence. So in the same way we need an effective "INTERNAL SECURITY SYSTEM" to be ever on guard, and be constantly dismissing disloyal, unfriendly, unproductive thoughts of fear and doubt, as well as NEGATIVE FEELINGS and NEGATIVE **PICTURES** that sneak into our minds.

With your LAF MAP you have a complete security guard system, internal and external. This system is to allow only those friendly and loyal **emotions** and **images** which have been tested, approved and accepted to enter.
The picture you create and hold in your mind as you relax and read your LAF material is to be that of your Security Guard, saluting and waving the LAF suggestions on in, directing them into the very inner offices of your mind.

Nathaniel Brandon, in "The Psychology of Self-Esteem", stated, "**The nature of his self-evaluation has profound effect on man's thinking process, emotions, desires, values and goals. It is the single most significant key to his behavior**." So check yourself closely. Have you found your negative PEP in your life? Make sure you have taken care of this most important step. By ourselves, on our own, most of us do not do a good job of thinking out and through our complex inner mind concerns and solving them. By following the LAF MAP you are being guided in doing just that.

Here are some steps to put your *security guard* to working properly:

     A.   Admit, acknowledge out loud on a recorder, what the real ROOT CAUSE is. "What NEED OR LACK am I TRYING to fulfill?"

     B.   Become more aware by WRITING IT DOWN. Put in your LAF ACHIEVMENT-BOOK everything you feel about your eating and about being overweight.

     (See: Recognizing your PREDOMINANT EMOTIOAL PROMPTERS.)

     C.   Confront, confess and keep admitting and confessing until you have completed this phase. Watch out for confessing only one part and then rationalizing that you have done the Job.

In writing your confession down, be careful and share this with no one on earth, except as mentioned herein, someone you love and trust, and you know loves and accepts you, and respects your confidentiality. Take plenty of time. There is a great advantage in this way. You can benefit greatly by sharing with that person. A wise minister, especially trained in counseling, or a priest or rabbi may be more objective. Stop NOW and do this phase when you have time to really relax and meditate.

Confess to God, the greatest counselor, while writing. Read it back and repeat the process until you have a knowing *feeling* that you have it all out.   Be keenly aware of what is revealed.

D. Declare it DONE!

You have the assurance that God forgives. Now it is time for you to accept God's acceptance. God loves you and forgives you, so LOVING YOURSELF MORE, you forgive yourself. You *let go*. Let go of all the negatives you have faced and confessed. Let go of all the real underlying root causes-*fear*, *insecurity*, resentment, bitterness, hostility and lack of <u>proper love</u>. Let go of the past. You can't change the past, but <u>*you can chance the NO W and the FUTURE!*</u>

CONGRATULATIONS! YOU HAVE NOW TAKEN VERY IMPORTANT ACTIONS ON YOUR LAF JOURNEY.

You realize the decisions that you have made in the past have brought you to your present condition. You can DECIDE – PRE-DECIDE --NOW to change.

LOVE AWAY FAT PROGRAM

CHECK THOSE WHICH APPLY TO YOU

NUMBER 1 TO 10 IF YOU WISH

AS IS NOW

I FEEL
   FAT
.   AWKWARD
   NERVOUS
   LIKE A NOBODY
   GUILTY
   EMBARRASSED
   TERRIBLE SELF—
   CONSCIOUS
   LAZY...TIRED
. . LIKE IT'S ALMOST
  A SELF-DESTRUCT
  LIKE I NEED TO
  DO SOMETHING

I DON'T FEEL.

LIKE A PERSON
LIKE I LIKE
   MYSELF ATTRACTIVE
LOVED
ENERGETIC

LAF GOAL IMAGE

I WANT TO FEEL
   PETITE
  ATTRACTVE
   SEXY
.   THIN
  FEMIN1NE
   SLENDER
   LIKE SOMEBODY
   HAPPY
   COMFORTABLE
GREAT ..TIDY
FULL OF LIFE
   CALM & RELAXED
   NEAT, •.NORMAL
   ENERGETIC

I WANT TO LOOK
SLIM .... YOUNG
.... GORGEOUS
  SHAPELY
  PRETTY
TRIM.... TALL

I LOOK LIKE
A POTATO SACK
FAT.... LIKE LARD
FAT AND FORTY

I DON'T LOOK
CLEAN AND NEAT
GOOD IN CLOTHES

I EAT
SWEETS....CHOCOLATE
BRADS ... POTATOES

I EAT
LIKE A HORSE
BETWEEN MEALS
HUGE AMOUNTS
FAST, TAKE BIG BITES
CHIPS....... ICE CREAM

I EAT WHEN
I AM ALONE
LONELY
BORED
I'M TIRED
I'M ANGRY
I'M UPSET
SAD .....HAPPY
FOOD IS THERE
I'M NOT REALLY
HUNGRY

I WANT TO LOOK
GOOD IN PANTS SUIT
STRONG
LOVELY
LOVEABLE
GOOD IN BIKINI

I WANT TO HAVE
MORE CONFIDENCE
A NICE APPEARANCE
A FLAT STOMACH
SELF DISCIPLINE

I WANT TO HAVE
FASHIONABLE
CLOTHES
AFFECTION
MY CHILDREN,
HUSBAND
PROUD OF ME
LOVE,
ROMANCE
SEX

I WANT
TO THINK MORE OF
MYSELF
TO ENJOY LOOKING AT
MYSELF IN THE MIRROR
TO DO MORE THINGS
TO GO PLACES

I…
LACK INITIATIVE
DISLIKE MYSELF
FIND CLOTHING HARD
   TO GET
HATE TO GO SHOPPING
AM CONSTANTLY
FIGHTING MYSELF
GET ANGRY WITH
MYSELF
AM ALWAYS A
DISAPPOINTMENT
AM NOT A DISCIPLINED
PERSON
AM DISGUSTED WITH
MYSELF
HATE MYSELF

I LOVE
CHOCOLATE
SWEETS
FOOD
ICE CREAM
IT
SEX

I WANT

PEOPLE TO THINK I'M
STRONG ENOUGH TO
CONTROL MYSELF

_

Remember to LOVE the person, but its O.K. to hate the hurt, the wrong, the deed that hurt you. It's all right to be angry, but not for twenty years! Be aware that you do not let that anger get turned inward and seethe. Being motivated, you have more and more perseverance. You keep at it until you are FREE! You have courage to stick with it. Commit yourself NOW to this LAF MAP, and as you carry out that commitment, YOU ARE GOING TO LOVE AND RESPECT YOURSELF MORE AND MORE!

COMPULSIVE EATING

"Less than two percent of the over-weight people have a glandular condition, and even then that condition is often partly the result of overeating instead of the other way around."

So states Dr. Eugene Scheimann.

Many parents, showing love as they know how, to their children, give them food, especially cookies, candy, ice cream, whenever the children experience hurt, physically or emotionally. Thus the person becomes conditioned to and programmed to cope with almost anything unpleasant by eating. Usually the eating is that of high calorie; high fat foods which are easily available. So when there is un-pleasantness, especially in the triune of LOVE, SEX and ROMANCE, that person behaves as he was programmed or scripted, and eats and eats and eats. Many overeaters structure their lives so that their secret is kept for the most part (except for the results). They "hide" things to eat, then they will practically go on a fast,- and then they will go on a binge.

RE-EDUCATION

A very important fact to face is that you can probably look great weighing a little more than you have considered as
Your desired weight!

Be realistic in setting your goal-image weight, not necessarily as you were at sixteen, or when you married, or as your favorite movie star.

LOVE, ROMANCE AND SEX

Dr. Scheimann also states, "As we have seen, the specific causes of real overweight are many and complex. But almost always for the American women, the fundamental cause is under-love.[3]

This applies to men too. LOVING YOURSELF MORE, you now embark on ways to bring more ROMANCE into your life. Let the triune of LOVE, ROMANCE and SEX become complete in your life, and then weight reduction follows naturally.

You look for and find things that bring interest, satisfaction, ROMANCE into your life! One can develop a love for a special project, or hobby. Refer to "IDEAS" in "HIGH, HAPPY AND HEALTHY."

As you have found out in Realization and Confessing, many of your activities run counter to achieving your objective, and fulfilling your real basic needs; so now you are paying more attention to your activities. Become aware of any negative activities. Ask yourself "If I love myself properly, will I continue in this activity?" Then repeat over and over, "I love myself, I love myself, I love myself. also use an appropriate LAF CARD and/or SCRIPT CARD such as number 20, 28, 29 or *53, 54,* 60, or 69.

The average American comes home from work, "relaxes", watches TV and eats! One sales executive told how he would have a carton of soft drinks and a can of pretzels by his chair, and while watching TV, would consume all in an evening! Another, a plumber, would stop by the ice cream parlor, buy a half-gallon of ice cream and do the same thing.

Many women tell me how they let TV take up their days and evenings. Whatever happened to romance? Husband and wife sit there, saying nothing of any consequence to each other except, "change the channel", perhaps without even a "Honey" or a "Please"! Why not change that to, "Honey, please turn off the TV, and come over here and turn me on!?"

The single person falls into the same trap. Why not, in God's name (I say it reverently), get up from in front of the TV, and find some rewording activity in which to get involved?

The way to an objective is through activities that lead to that objective. The more LOVE, ROMANCE and SEX you can involve in these activities, the more effective they will be in moving you toward your goal image. I don't mean once a month or once a week. Why not every day?

With LOVING AWAY FAT, you find yourself modifying your attitude about food and how you use it. You are becoming more and more aware of the misuse and thus find yourself changing that into a more satisfying behavior that brings pleasing results.

You also modify your thinking about exercise, realizing that *EXERCISE ALONE* cannot keep you at your goal-weight and shape. You realize it can help tone you up, make you feel better, look better and perk up your self-concept. You'll love yourself more.

You also modify your eating behavior. The cues, the situations, the stimuli that in the past caused you to eat and/or overeat no longer entice you. You are FREE. No longer does TV and food go together; nor do commercials appeal to you. It's easier and easier to drive right on past the quick food drive-ins. Remember every time that you are tempted, that there many people out there who are succeeding in their weight reduction and control. You are one of them! Your inner mind (your subconscious) maintains a constant vigilance and the LIBERATING POWER OF LOVE comforts you. LOVING YOURSELF MORE, look for ways to bring more interest, more romance into your work, your social life, your family life.

You are to develop a dynamic, active attitude toward LOVE. Refuse to follow the herd of those inactive TV lovers and begin pursuing ROMANCE.

Dr. Albert Schweitzer puts it this way, "We are all so much together, but we are all dying of loneliness."[2] How do you keep from dying of loneliness?

Leave the self-pity party, and start putting ROMANCE into your life. A person who has his or her "antenna" up, who is mentally and emotionally ready to receive love, and has the desire "tuned in" for the triune of LOVE, ROMANCE and SEX relationship, will find it drawn to him or her.

If you are "fat", don't wait until you are thin to start on your adventure of ROMANCE. Start putting up your antenna NOW, TODAY. Pre-decide. Make the decision NOW that you ARE romantic. If you don't know how, watch some of' those who do, or find a wholesome book on the subject. Maybe there is one on "Love, Romance, and Sex". IF not, there should be. Perhaps you can write it!

Remember a woman may FEEL LOVED by a man showing affection, and without sex, and more fulfilled than when having sex without affection. Neither is as fulfilling as when having LOVE, ROMANCE and SEX! Since we gain so much pleasure, so much satisfaction through our mouths, let us look for a moment at the many activities available to us to obtain more oral pleasure.

Satisfaction and satiety.

Dr. Scheimann continues: "For there are numerous oral-centered or oral triggered outlets that are not merely sexual. What of the wonderful hugs and kisses involved in caring for children? This is a key area for both married and single folks. So is affection in general as shown through a kiss." [3]

For married folks, how long do you keep the spirit or the wedding vows -LOVE, HONOR etc.?

I know marrieds in their seventies and eighties who are still romantic, AND sexually satisfied! When is the last time you laid a really good kiss on your mate? With some relatively young marriages I've observed, there is little more than a peck of a kiss when leaving or coming home from work, or even after being separated for several days! There is little or absolutely no affection shown for days on end. Even in sex there is not a single kiss, No wonder one feels unfulfilled, hungry. They are starved for LOVE, ROMANCE and SEX.

Remember, if one has sex only, there is still something lacking. So they search for something and put the closest, most convenient things into the oral cavity. And that usually is something like a candy bar or those easy carbohydrates in the cabinet, refrigerator or snack machine.

"Sweets for the sweet", and the most enjoyed in the world is chocolate!

Do not wait for the time when you will be trim, and beautiful. Act as if you are, right now! Then you will wake up some morning and find that you do not have to "act as if'.

THE PLUMP TEENAGER

Here is a word to the plump teenager. Adults also can benefit from these principles. Not loving herself enough, she has to lie to herself and others pretending not to be interested in boys. She then substitutes other activities, with eating at the top at the list. Any other activities are likely to be of a sedentary nature. Not loving herself enough, she separates herself further from those with whom she really needs to feel togetherness. She likes food. Food tastes good. Food brings pleasure; and without romance in her life, *food* becomes her main daily pleasure. Note the time she does most of it. It is when she comes home from, school and at night, even, after a big dinner and couldn't possibly he hungry, except BEING hungry for LOVE and ROMANCE. Then a vicious circle sets in. She doesn't have romance in her life because she is plump. She *thinks*, "What's the use? Why not really have pleasure and eat, eat all I want?" **But it doesn't satisfy**.

Then a misuse of love takes over –resentfulness, bitterness, and rebellion. Keeping it to herself she thinks subconsciously, if not consciously, "They can't keep me from this enjoyment." And the cycle continues.

She thinks "food', looks forward to food, while other girls are thinking "boys", and looking forward to dates and other satisfying activities. The process does not bring long-lasting satisfaction; so she eats more and more, getting fatter and fatter. Food tastes good, but satisfying only when in the mouth, just temporarily. So the pattern perpetuates itself.

LAUFF

LOVE AWAY UNWANTED FAT FOREVER!!

PART II

INNER MIND POWER AFFIRMATIONS

Use the TOGETHERNESS EXERCISE before reading the
INNER MTND POWER AFFIRMATIONS following.
<u>READ   ONCE A DAY FOR FIVE WEEKS AND FIVE DAYS</u>.
Then read as often as you wish for reinforcement.

For emphasis, some material from Part I is repeated in Part II
as INNER MIND POWER AFFIRMATIONS.

READ AND
LOVE AWAY FAT!

45

LOVE

YOU CAN'T <u>SAVE</u> LOVE!
YOU CAN'T SPEND LOVE!
YOU CAN ONLY SHARE IT -
YOU SHARE LOVE AND
STILL HAVE IT!
YOU "GIVE" LOVE AND
LOVE IS MULTIPLIED!
YOU GIVE
AND GET TN LOVE.

OTHER PEPs and PIMs

What are some of your other possible PEP's and PIM's? Is the child-self within wanting to lay the blame elsewhere, rather than taking on the mature adult-self attitude of assuming RESPONSIBILITY? Many times people try to balance the guilt in their lives with blame. "Blame them!" LOVE is assuming responsibility for self.

Also check to see if there is any tendency for the child-self to have a pity-party, wanting others to feel sorry for him. Is the child-self feeling dependent, crying out to the adult-self, "Please take care of me"? Check this closely when you seem unhappy. SEE: "RECOGNIZING YOUR PEPS AND PIMS", and study: "List of True Basic Needs" to help you understand better YOUR REAL LACK

As you look at all these reasons for self-punishment, for dependency, for self-pity, and feeling helpless, you clearly see that the very things* being used to bring love do NOT bring *love, security* or happiness. With the LAF MAP, your adult-self learns more acceptable and successful ways to achieve these needs. *("Things" can be smoking tobacco, marijuana, etc., drinking, taking drugs, promiscuous sex, and on and on.) These "things" DO NOT bring about a good self-image, including self-respect, self-trust, self-worth, love, and acceptance, success and happiness!

You now may have come to the conclusion that self-punishment does not relieve guilt permanently. It relieves only temporarily if at all. Thus the *reason* for the continuing in the fallacy. The fact is that self-punishment brings on more guilt and thus tends to set up a vicious cycle: more anger, more guilt, and more punishment and on and on! Like the emotion of fear, guilt should be only a fleeting feeling in your life. "Perfect love casts out fear"[1], and that same love, love of God, can cast your guilt "as far as the East is from the West."[2] The Bible also tells us, "If we confess our sins, He (God) is faithful and just, and will forgive our sins and cleanse us from all unrighteousness."[3] Guilt can be handled - done away with by confessing and then *accepting* forgiveness.

"OK. OK", you say, "So I'm angry, feel guilty, and I'm punishing myself. What can I do about it? How can I stop?" First, you now realize that it is absolutely right and important, even crucial, that you feel guilty about some things. This is mentally, emotionally, and spiritually healthy.

Second, you realize that it is useless to feel guilty about trivia, like, "What will others think?", or certain things that "Mom or "Dad" said were "bad". They could be bad, but just because they said so doesn't make it so.

Third, you do not have to punish yourself for ANYTHING, especially for how you feel!

Don't try to play God. At the same time, realize That God doesn't want to punish you either. "But God, who is rich in mercy, out of the great love with which he loved us"~ is forbearing, "not wishing that any should perish, but that ALL should reach repentance. After confessing, is there anything you can do to make amends, to restore relationships back to normal? "First be reconciled to your brother", then come to the Altar of' Confession (to God). (See "HANDLING OFFENCES" for additional references on this subject.)

Become aware of what you are really doing when you punish yourself. By "mutilating" your body with *fat*, you are living an illusion, thinking that self-punishment will purge you of guilt. The way to handle guilt properly is to face reality and realize you can be FREE OF GUILT and FREE OF THOSE EXTRA POUNDS and BE HAPPY!

Now love yourself in a healthy way. You realize no one is perfect. Be thankful you are as nearly perfect as you are and that you are acceptable to God. So loving yourself more, you accept yourself. You make amends and accept the forgiveness of God and others. You accept God's acceptance of you. You accept forgiveness from yourself.

Loving yourself more, you accept yourself as you are <u>NOW</u> no matter what or how you feel or how you look. Again, say over and over and over, "I LIKE MYSELF, I LIKE MYSELF, I LIKE MYSELF--".

Then you find that you move forward to becoming loving, lovable and lovely (handsome)!

LAF, LOVE IS THE CHANGING POWER

You are to be congratulated for loving yourself caring enough for yourself (and others) to take the time and effort to get into this "Love Away Fat" MAP..

You are not to regard this "MAP" as a "side road," "detour," a temporary plan or gimmick in your way of living.
Regard it as a turn-around, a "legal U-turn." You have discovered that you have been going in the wrong direction. You simply make a 180-degree turn-around, and now you are going away from failure to success - a way that is leading you home, home free!

Go through books on psychology, sociology, anthropology, etc. Think back over your years in elementary school, high school and college. How many courses, how many books did you study on LOVE? Isn't that fantastic! The greatest of all is LOVE, and you probably never had one class in it. Oh, we have been spoon-fed bits and pieces in Bible school and in sermons. How often have we heard sermons specifically on "Love," "How To love," or "How To Love Yourself Better?!" Of course we learn from parents by following their examples of living, but they may have been
stumbling along too.

Using LAF, you can be assured. God has promised it. Jesus said so. You are what you are as a result of your thoughts, especially in the inner mind. "As a man thinketh in his heart, so is he"[1] You can be what you want to be as a result of this "Loving Yourself More" way.

You realize LOVE is the Changing Power. You are a loving person. You love yourself. You are doing good things for yourself You are kind to yourself and do kind things to and
49

for yourself. As you love yourself more, you are in **better** position to love others more. You show your love for God by doing good and kind things for others and for yourself

As you love yourself more, your faith is becoming stronger. You are more confident and self-assured. You believe more and more in yourself each day, and your belief in God is stronger.

Because of your love for yourself, you accept yourself as God created you, as God intends you to be. You know that He loves you and wants the best for you and yours. You realize "God is not finished with you yet." You are a maturing, loving person.

Not only are you going to find it easy to read and accept these affirmations, these scripts at least once each day, you will be reminded of them many times in between.

With your LAF MAP you have a complete *Security Guard* system, internal and external. This system is to allow the entering of only those friendly and loyal emotions and images which have been tested, approved and accepted.

The picture you create and hold in your mind, as you relax and read, is to be that of your Security Guard, saluting and waving the LAF affirmations on in, directing them into the very inner offices of your mind.

Also remember, being motivated, you have more and more perseverance. You keep at it until you are FREE! You have courage to stick with it. Commit yourself NOW to this LAF MAP, and as you carry out that commitment, YOU ARE GOING TO LOVE AND RESPECT YOURSELF MORE AND MORE!

If you go to the refrigerator or the cabinet or the coke machine, or food vendor, you hear the LAF affirmations in your mind. You see them in action and reality; you hear them; you feel them. When you smell food, the picture-affirmations flash onto the screen of your mind. When you hear others on TV or at work mentioning food or drink, you experience comforting reassurances that result from these affirmations. Cues that in the past had triggered your eating and/or drinking practices now remind you of how secure in love you feel. The cues bring to mind your recognition of love, as it should be. Loving yourself more, you pre-decide what you are going to do in all the various, previously troublesome situations.

You use the "Mental Movie Technique" to practice your LOVE-SELF-MORE principles. You do this in advance, thus preparing yourself to make the proper response under any circumstance. You are prepared for all kinds of negative situations. You are fortified from within, *secure* in your deep inner love for yourself. Infinite love envelops you, protects you, pacifies you, holds you, calms you, comforts you, *and secures* you.

You feel contented and satisfied. You feel the comfort of deep warm love surrounding you like a warm cozy blanket on a cold night. Infinite love permeates your mind-brain-body and your very soul. Love is creating on invisible shield about you. Thoughts opposed to your GOAL-IMAGE cannot penetrate this SHIELD OF LOVE.
You feel *safe, secure and serene.*

You love and protect your physical self as a loving and caring parent loves and protects a child. Your LOVE disciplines lovingly to let new, acceptable, and good patterns of behavior develop.

Each of us is accountable for one's self. Your love for yourself strengthens you in your accountability. Your love bears fruits of responsibility and self-care. These in turn reinforce your love. You are letting this positive love-circle become stronger and stronger. As a consequence, your healthy self-concept is that of a very confident and self-assured person.

Your acceptance of God's Love brings to you the assurance that *you* **belong.** Love brings a *belonging feeling* in place of a longing-for feeling- a full and satisfied feeling instead of emptiness that won't go away. Love brings satisfaction and contentment, instead of discontentment. You feel accepted. You feel approved. You feel a sense of worth.

As time goes on and your weight comes down to your best love-image, your love sustains you. You develop new habits of thought, new behavior.

You feel worthy! You feel competent! You feel confident!

HOW CAN YOU HELP YOURSELF? How can you cope with the painful or unpleasant feelings, and also enjoy happy feelings?

Here and now you make the DECISION to inspire yourself to become your better self, to lift yourself up. You can do it with this LAF MAP!

Talking to yourself by name (your other name, middle name, etc., you say "We're together on this; I'm for you, and you, (other name), are for me! We choose to do just those things that make us feel good about ourselves!"

As you follow this LAF routine, you are more and more aware of the things in your life that help you (both of you) to feel good and to appreciate yourselves more.

You find it easier and easier each day, as you practice these thought patterns, to see yourself as you truly are within. You are friendly with your inner-self. You converse with your inner-self by name, and become aware of what you have been doing to keep you from reaching your objective – becoming your better self, not perfect self. No one is perfect, and you accept that fact. You are more and more aware of any of the ways that you put yourself down. You have made the DECISION: That is not for you. Say it, "That's not for me!" You start RIGHT NOW doing just those things that cause you to feel good about yourself, that give you so much greater satisfaction and pleasure.

You are keenly aware of your fine qualities and your achievements, those of the past, and in the NOW, and in the FUTURE. When you achieve something that you feel good about, you are going to dwell on it awhile. You let it enter- and re-enter your *inner-mind,* You enjoy it. You relish it. You compliment yourself, and are lavish in your praise for yourself. You recognize the achievement, giving yourself "stars."

You accept compliments from others with a simple "Thank you," but you internalize the compliment and continue to let it boost you over a longer period of time. Keep a journal of them, "TRIBUTES" in your LAF ACHIEVEMENTR-BOOK. Refer to them often. You, in turn compliment yourself and let the good, warm feeling remain within you.

Loving yourself more, you appreciate yourself more and more. If you fail a moment or a day on your program of progress, you merely look on that as a learning experience. You do not scold or curse yourself or whop yourself over the head! You are kind, forgiving and accepting. You then find it easier to get right back on track, remembering the times you were successful, and these times get longer and longer. Loving yourself, you know it is OK to be successful over a longer and longer period.

Loving yourself more and more, you find it easier and easier to feel good about yourself.

Loving yourself more, you have compassion for yourself. When you are "bad" or feel bad, you ask your-self such questions as "Do I really enjoy feeling this way?" "What will the feeling accomplish?" "Will it make me love myself more?" Then you find it easier and easier to do good and kind things for yourself that will cause you to feel good inside. You love your-self more. You do more good things for yourself; then you love yourself more. You are building a positive love upward spiral.

Loving yourself more, you are aware of the inner compulsion to procrastinate to put off those things you know logically you need to do and should do, but don't want to do NOW. When this process of thinking starts, it is your hypnotic cue which reminds you to do what you know is right for you. You then find yourself more and more automatically following through. Thus you avoid the putdowns of; "I'm disgusted with myself." Or "I hate myself for not doing those things!" Etc., etc. At the same time, you have good feelings of achievement; and recognizing these; you compliment yourself and relish the good feelings that follow. You love yourself more!

As Cecil Osborne points out in his book, "You're in Charge;" "You are in charge of your decisions, your choices, and your ultimate fate. The initiative is yours."
As you love your-self more, you accept this responsibility and, along with it, the exhilarating feeling that comes from knowing, "I'm in charge! I'm in control."

"Looking inward," "thinking of self," "loving self"-these and other phrases about "self" may seem selfish to some people, but hear this out, Dale Galloway in "How to Feel Like A Somebody Again," says,

53

"Self-love is the direct opposite of self-centeredness."[2]

"Doing what makes you feel good about yourself is really the opposite of self-indulgence," Mildred Newman and Bernard Berkowitz, practicing psychoanalysts, state in their book, "How To Be Your Own Best Friend," "It means satisfying your whole self"[3]

As you love yourself more, you really are not denying yourself the good things of life. When you love yourself properly, you can truly deny yourself. You are free to surrender to God and others, without fear of losing yourself, without fear of giving up your will, your ego. Rather than being selfish and trying to hold onto, you let go. You are FREE TO BE, to receive, to give, to RECEIVE LOVE, to GIVE LOVE, to LIVE FULLY THAT HIGH, HEALTHY AND HAPPY LIFE.

As you follow your LAF MAP, which is your "MY ACHIEVEMENT PLAN," you are benefiting more and more. You are achieving a better self-image. You have a better self-concept. Thus you have more love to share! As you love yourself more, you enjoy a new FREEDOM. You are free to do as you have in the past but you are also FREE NOT to act in that negative way. You are FREE to make that RIGHT DECISION. You now act in a positive way. You pre-decide certain issues, what you are going to do in certain situations. Then when the temptations arise, you find that you don't have to fight the battles; you simply carry out the decisions you've already made! There is no "wishing I could," or "sure would be good, but I'd better not," It is simply a "NO THANK YOU" attitude.

You feel good inwardly, carrying out the responsibility you have assumed. You are encouraged. You do things and say things to encourage yourself'
YOU LOVE YOURSELF MORE!
54

Loving yourself more, you have more faith, more confidence in yourself, more of a positive attitude. You thus love yourself EVEN more, and move upward in a positive success spiral. When negatives start to come into your mind, these act as "posthypnotic cues," which remind you to immediately replace the negatives with POSITIVES. AND IT IS SO

When such statements as "I can't help it" or "I don't have willpower" come into your mind, at the very least, change them to: "In the PAST, I couldn't -" This will cue to your inner mind and encourage you to do good and kind things for yourself. Treat yourself, as you want to be and should be, not as you have been! YOU LOVE YOURSELF MORE AND MORE!

Your having a genuine desire to do certain things is God's way of telling you that you can be a success in that desire. Therefore, you focus only on your Positive Predominant Image Motivator for your objective ~your new self-image.

LOVE IS THE CHANGING POWER!

You are letting God's LOVE flow into you and permeate every mind-brain cell, so that as you love yourself more, you also find you are loving others more, and in turn loving yourself more and loving God more! And then something wonderful has happened; you find that you don't have to *TRY* anymore. You are in that positive upward success spiral; SUCCESS BUILDING UPON SUCCESS.
YOU LOVE YOURSELF MORE AND MORE AND MORE!!

You accept the fact that people resist change. They especially resist change in a habit they have become comfortable with- even though it is not leading them toward their real objective. Accepting and acknowledging that fact (confessing it), and making a DECISION to turn in a different direction in

your life, calls into your life a great INNER-MIND-POWER that moves obstacles aside, LETTING you proceed toward your objective, "LOVING THYSELF"!
YOU LOVE YOURSELF MORE!

LOVE IS THE LIBERATING POWER!

In "Living, Loving and Learning," Dr. Leo Buscaglia puts it this way: "Stop working against yourself. Let's get away from this frozen self. Remember that you are a holy thing. You are God's gift. So give birth to yourself.   Allow you out.
Get rid of all those self-defeating ideas, self-defeating ideas about others that keep you and me from coming together. Learn to trust again. **Learn to forgive**.
"You can make the decision today to drop these crazy, self-defeating ideas, and to be all that God intended you to be, which is the least thing you can do for God."~

You realize that your NEGATIVE PREDOMINANT EMOTIONAL PROMPTER and NEGATIVE PREDOMINANT IMAGE MOTIVATOR may have been fitting and perfectly OK for you and the situation in times past-even in a positive way. As time and circumstances have changed, you recognize the negative effects **now**, and you are WILLING BOTH CONSCIOUSLY AND SUBCONSCIOUSLY TO CHANCE.

You realize that you do not have to FEEL that you have been "wrong" all this time. However if you were, or *feel* that you really were wrong, you can be assured that you have forgiveness and freedom from that guilt, simply by reaching out for it. Feeling sorry and wanting to get rid of the guilt and the guilty feeling, you simply admit your wrongs to God, who "is faithful and just, and will forgive our sins and cleanse us from ALL unrighteousness."[5]

"So if the Son makes you free, you will be free indeed."[6] First, you now realize that it is absolutely right and important, even crucial, that you feel guilty about some things. This is mentally, emotionally, and spiritually healthy. Secondly you realize that it is useless to feel guilty about trivia, like, "What will others think?" or certain things that "Mom" or "Dad" said were "bad." They could be bad, but just because they said so doesn't make it so. Thirdly, you do not have to punish yourself for ANYTHING, especially for how you *feel!* Don't try to play God. At the same time, realize that God doesn't want to punish you either. "But God, who is rich in mercy, out of the great love with which he loved us"[4] is forbearing, "not wishing that any should perish, but That ALL should reach repentance."[5]

After confessing, is there anything you can do to make amends, to restore relationships back to normal? "First be reconciled to your brother,"[6] then come to the Altar of Confession (to God).

Become aware of what you are really doing when you punish yourself. By "mutilating" your body with fat, you are living in an illusion, thinking that self-punishment will purge you of guilt. The way to handle guilt properly is to face reality and realize you can be FREE OF GUILT and THOSE EXTRA POUNDS and BE HAPPY!
Now love yourself in a healthy way. You realize no one is perfect. Be thankful you are as nearly perfect as you are and that you are acceptable to God. So loving yourself, you accept yourself. You make amends and accept the forgiveness of God and others.

You accept God's acceptance of you. You accept forgiveness from yourself.

Loving yourself more, you accept your-self as you are NOW. no matter what you feel or how you look. Then you find that you move forward to becoming loving, lovable and lovely (handsome)!

It is OK to change. It is thrilling to change. It's exciting! You get more satisfaction and pleasure from changing.

Guilt is one negative PEP we all have at times and, at least subconsciously feel that we must be punished. Guilt calls for punishment! But you now realize, as you think on this, you do not have to balance guilt with punishment. You can be FREE of BOTH GUILT and PUNISHMENT. God has promised a way for this! Believe it and accept his love into your inner mind, your heart.

Declare it DONE! You have the assurance that God Forgives. Now it is time for you to accept God's acceptance.

God loves you and forgives you, so LOVING YOURSELF, you forgive yourself. You let go. Let go of all the negatives you have faced and confessed. Let go of all the real underlying root causes, fear, insecurity, resentment, bitter-ness, hostility, lack of proper love, etc. Let go of the past. You can't change the past, but you can change the NOW and the FUTURE!

Now take a big breath and with God's forgiveness, symbolically exhale all guilt. GOD has expelled all guilt and thus there is no need for punishment! Loving yourself, you accept this forgiveness, this freedom and cancel all self-punishment.

AND IT IS SO!

POSI-PEP, PUNISHMENT

As you search your inner mind for your PEP, you may find, like some that you really look on punishment as a Posi-PEP. Punishment, to many, unfortunately, is associated with being cared for, or "loved." As a child punishment or indifference is all some received, and a significant part of what others received from well-meaning parents. Punishment, a child can take, but not indifference (lack of love). So ask yourself, have I been one of those who wanted punishment? Your inner mind may have said punishment was the best thing that happened to you. Some have learned to regard it as a reward! It was togetherness as opposed to loneliness that you may have experienced otherwise, and dreaded! You may have felt rejected except when punished. It was getting attention. It was filling a lack in your life. A basic permanent human need is to *feel loved* and accepted. As a loving p a r e n t   s e l f, you are NOT going to allow yourself to punish yourself, trying to fulfill any lack in your life. You are not going to punish yourself with unsightly FAT! Neither do you have to play the role of a punishing parent to your child-self.

As an adult, you put away that childhood and now enjoy your independence and the fun and joy that comes from being your adult-self

Loving your adult-self more, you now can really *receive love from others more,* because you can give it more. You let it flow through you; you receive it with joy.

"Make LOVE your AIM."!

59

You now realize as an adult that you can, in fact, enjoy aloneness at times. When you are alone, when your family is gone, you still feel self-assured, self-sufficient and LOVED. *You feel secure.* You do good things for yourself. You are kind to your adult-self. You feel more independent. You stand on your own feet. You have adult-parent confidence. Your child-self feels *safe and secure,* as one should feel when loved and cared for as a child.

Loving yourself more, you couple your inner feelings --your emotions with the intellect, the logic of your outer mind. You use your inner mind *imagination* along with your *will* of your outer-self, your conscious mind. You are using everything available to you to help you tap more and more of that tremendous potential within. Ask yourself: what is in it for ME?

The REWARDS are GREAT!

You are aware of what, when and where your behavior does not help you achieve the goal-image you really want. Loving yourself more, you welcome the change to new habits of thoughts, new behavior. This new behavior moves you away from the so-called satisfying behavior of the past with unsatisfactory results, and moves you to pleasing behavior NOW and in the FUTURE. This leads you to satisfying BENEFITS-- a self-loving, appreciating self-image of being your better self. So now, LOVING YOURSELF MORE, you let go of past debilitating behavior and welcome the change that comes into your life.

You more and more easily give way to new more satisfactory actions for yourself in the now and the future. You are free to change! You are looking forward with pleasurable anticipation to changing into the better you.. With many, the Nega-PEP is a response to some offense by someone or some situation in early childhood, perhaps not realizing the anger or other negative feeling is still there. You now take a good adult view of what is happening in your life. You realize what unresolved anger does to your life, not to the offender; your internalized anger does not hurt them. It hurts you. Remember to LOVE the person, but it's Okay to hate the hurt, the wrong, the deed that hurt you. It's all right to be angry, but not for twenty years! Be aware that you do not let that anger get turned inward and seethe. LOVING YOURSELF MORE, you LET GO of any anger-. You let go and FORGIVE! You LET GO. You are Free to LET GO. You take a trip by the mental trash can and dump any resentment, bitterness, any grievance, and any revengeful attitude. NOW, you are FREE of that weighting-down load. (Study the Hurt Map.)

LOVING YOURSELF MORE, you realize as an adult, you are FREE to please YOURSELF. Please God and please you! You do not have to please your parents, your brothers or sisters, or teachers, etc., in the same manner as you did as a child. You are not small and dependent as you were as a child. As an adult, you are pleasing yourself and are not held back. You can make your own decisions and do your own thing within God's will, not theirs. You have courage to move out of the womb of childhood *security and* safety.

You enjoy the rewards, the sense of accomplishment and confidence that can come only with the broad adventurous actions of adulthood and of the continuously maturing adult-self.

LOVING YOURSELF MORE, you assert yourself. As you do so, you are not diminishing another, especially your parents and family, or the child you were. You are FREE to be HIGH, HAPPY AND HEALTHY! You now know you are not putting down your parents by lifting yourself up. You are not destroying their image, or your own earlier-self, by building up your NOW-SELF and FUTURE-SELF, your better self-image. You are building on those strengths. You are not denying the real needs of the two, three, five year old child you were —and who is still a part of you. You LOVE that child-part of you, and are caring, considerate, and *forgiving*.

You now find it easier and easier to face such feelings, deal with them, and move through them as you would move through a door to a powerful, yet beautiful life on the other side. You are opening that door NOW to a HAPPY and HEALTHY life, a more interesting life, a more exciting life!
You are closing the door behind to the fear of disapproval, fear of failure, fear of hurting, and fear of defeat.

By reading this LAF MAP, you have made the DECISION TO DO IT NOW not tomorrow or the next week, but RIGHT NOW! You are developing more patience, more perseverance, and more determination. LOVING YOURSELF MORE, you assert yourself more, and you feel encouraged. You encourage yourself! You have more courage and more and more confidence.
You feel reassured

Again, remember that as you LOVE YOURSELF MORE, you are free to fail now and then- to fall backward. You just look on these slips as learning experiences, and get right back on track. You have confidence to do those things that move you toward your goal-image. You have courage and confidence to change, to let go of the debilitating habits. You are letting go.

You are learning to let go of the Nega-PEP, and are inspired by your POSI-PEP.

LOVING YOURSELF MORE, you are free to use your child-like imagination and visualize or picture yourself as you really want to be and should be. It becomes easy this way. Then you come to realize that all you may have thought you had to give up is of little consequence in light of the tremendous and exciting life you are going to have.

LOVING YOURSELF MORE, every day, every moment of the time, you are going to be aware, keenly aware of any of the old debilitating activities. You are attentive to any actions that do not move you toward your goal-image. If you start to stray, you ask yourself such questions as "What good can this possibly do *me?* Why am I eating this fattening food?" You then become aware of your POSI-PEP and/or your POSI-PIM within. More than likely you readily recognize its relationship to LOVING YOURSELF. Then the temptation melts away and vanishes. The Nega-PEPs and Nega-PIMs are dissipated!

IDENTIFICATION

might be your Nega-PIM now. It was your Posi-PIM as a child. You have identified with your parents. That is where you first developed your identity.

Now as an adult, you have your own identity. You are not lost without them. Now you realize the negative habits you want to change may be a result of identifying with a loved one. You love and admire them; so you not only strive to be like their noble characteristics, but subconsciously take on the negatives as well. These are Negative-Predominant IMAGE Motivators for your adult-self. You now choose a Positive-Predominant IMAGE-Motivator to replace that negative motivator. It is **your own**.

You are careful to observe any behavior of yours that has taken on the negative characteristics of any other person. You are aware of any imitations or identifying with your mother or father image that does not <u>at this time</u>, serve your love-self-more-image.

You are becoming more consciously aware of the parson(s) or principle(s) that you have been referring to as a "standard." Who is your Standard of Comparison? Remember, as E. Stanley Jones pointed out, "If you surrender to anything this side of God, it will let you down."[1] So set your own standard, with God's help. Realize that even when one says, "I am NOT going to be like (name of person)," or "I'm not going to do like ", he or she is still using that "Standard of Comparison," and tends to BECOME LIKE THAT PERSON.

Therefore be very careful of the standard you choose.

You visualize yourself as you want to be. You are becoming what you want to be! You are self-assured, self-sufficient, self-loved, and thus you can share more love with others around you.

You love and protect your physical self as a loving and caring parent loves and protects a child. Your LOVE disciplines lovingly to let new, acceptable, and good patterns of behavior develop.

Imagine that a small refuge child has been placed in your care. This child knows nothing about the eating of proper foods. Now ask yourself the questions, "Would I give to this child or allow this child to eat the 'junk food' that I eat? Would I allow this child to eat all the sweets and fat foods that I eat? Would I allow this child to eat the amounts that I eat?"

As a loving and caring "PARENT-SELF", you now show the some loving concern for the "CHILD-SELF" within you. Your baby-self and child-self learned certain techniques to experience love and security. Those techniques were a matter of survival to you then. You learned to love and be loved, to manipulate to survive, at least in your child-mind. Now as a self-loving adult, you put away childlike attitudes and techniques. Loving yourself, you pay close attention to your adult-self and your child-self, looking, listening, and feeling. You are more aware of what is going on in your inner mind, your inner self. Then it becomes easy and automatic to follow a self-loving mode of living, taking nothing into your body to mar or scar it, or to load it down.

You seek only to nurture, nourish, and cherish it. As you exercise even a little nurturing, you start the upward spiral into a positive success cycle.
You build larger successes upon larger successes.

Even if you slip a little in your upward success spiral, you look at it for what it is, just a slip, not a return to the old self-diminishing, negative, downward spiral. You have broken that one, and you accept the fact that your upward spiral has its bumps and slumps. That is just part of the challenge, the journey, the adventure, the good times, and happiness that continue to increase the farther up you go. You make the conscious and subconscious DECISION NOW to take the upward spiral. You have PRE-DECIDED. You take charge of that child-self You let go of any childish ways; you are learning to let go. You are learning to take charge, to take hold of yourself as a loving parent takes charge of a misbehaving child. The child-self will understand a firm "No!".

YOU HAVE CONTROL.

You make the decision over and over, and then one day you find you don't have to make it. Your LAF-MAP WAY has become a habit! Then it is automatic and easy!

Along the way, the child-self within may throw a few tantrums, may fight the changes, may act as if the child-self is fighting for survival. You are loving, accepting, non-judgmental, forgiving, and moving on past the tantrums. Now you realize the way for the child-self to survive is to let it grow up into the adult intended, putting away childish things. As the Bible states, "Do not be childish in your thinking; but in thinking be mature." You have patience and perseverance. As negatives come into your mind, you change them into positives. You love yourself and build up your adult-self emotionally and spiritually. You compliment your adult-self for every positive change. You are lavish in your praise. You show real love.

"MAKE LOVE YOUR AIM"

Not only do you forgive the child-self for the occasional misbehaving now, but you also forgive the child-self for all the bad in the early years. The "bad" may be real or imagined. Either way let it go. You are letting go. You realize sometimes you have to be firmer than at other times, BUT ALWAYS LOVING.

YOU LOVE YOURSELF MORE! AND IT IS SO.

HYPNOTIC-SUGGESTIONS-AFFIRMATIONS

SELF-LOVE; SELF-ESTEEM; SELF-ACCEPTANCE; SELF-APPROVAL.

You have a legitimate, acceptable desire to attain your WORTHY, WORTHWHILE OBJECTIVE, You have a healthy inner drive to achieve your goal set for and by you. You realize that you have to compete only with yourself. You are developing this habit of competing only with yourself. You have a sensible drive to achieve, not to excel or "beat" someone else, but to satisfy your own self; that which God would want for you.

You do not have to compensate for feelings of inferiority. You are a unique person.
You only have to compete with YOUR previous achievements.
You have a quiet determination to surpass your previous achievements.

You do not go out of your way to win the approval of others-anyone. Your strong sense of identity gives you a good feeling of being of help to others, being needed and, at the same time, not having an excessive need to be needed.

You know you can, and may say, "No," when conditions of the situation warrant it.
You feel no guilt for having said, "No."

You are a self-accepting person.
YOU GIVE LOVE, AND YOU ACCEPT LOVE. You are sensitive to the feelings and needs of others; yet you do not overly respond. You are never hypercritical, sarcastic, or overly sensitive. People who are self-rejecting often criticize others and project their own self-rejection onto them by saying sarcastic things and/or by showing other forms of hostility. Loving yourself and being self-accepting, self-approving, you guard against such tactics by being aware of any such behavior. You quickly replace it with the "I love you" thought projection.
Looking at the person, just mentally and silently say, "I love you."

The Love-Vision Technique penetrates the coldest of attitudes and melts walls of hostility.

Learning to love yourself more and more, you realize that it is OK to have anger in your life in certain situations. Jesus, the Son of God, did, and so did some of His followers. Loving yourself and loving others, you handle your anger in a constructive, creative way. You are more and more aware of how to express it appropriately. You carefully suppress it at times, but you are very, very careful and mindful of any denying of anger, of repressing it, especially of turning it inward. The wisdom and power within you guide you in handling anger in a loving constructive way.

You live in the here and now. You realize you cannot change bad history, and you do not keep going over it. You also realize you can change your NOW and the future. Loving yourself as a worthy person, you have contentment and satisfaction. You live in the present, setting worthwhile objectives for the future.

Instead of depending on others to "make" you happy, you give of yourself to others, making yourself happy, and finding that love flows back to you. Loving yourself more, you seek ways to complete your objective, your goals, your hopes, your dreams. You compliment yourself upon every achievement and accept compliments lovingly. You are glad when others achieve and prosper. You are glad when YOU achieve and prosper. You refrain from judging yourself. *You forgive* yourself. You recognize love within you, and let it flow through you to others.

YOU ACT ON YOUR LOVE!

Food, in itself, that is, food without LOVE can never bring satiety, that full satisfaction, while inner anxieties remain. If you can alleviate the anxiety, the lack of love, great! IF you absolutely cannot, if it is completely beyond your control, you can resolve, pre-decide NOW and forever, that FOOD is not going to be used to *try*. It has not worked in the past. It will not do it in the now, or in the future! Various activities can be used, but never over eating and drinking!

IF you agree, nod your head and say, "Yes, I resolve to use food only for nutrition. And since it is for nutrition only, I eat sparingly, slowly, simply and properly.
AND IT IS SO!"

Loving yourself more, you find it easier and easier to create LAF activities- LOVE activities that express your love for yourself and to others. You contact the Spirit of Wisdom within, bringing forth new patterns of pleasing and satisfying activities.
ALL OF LIFE IS MORE INTERESTING AND EXCITING. As you love yourself more, you can and do love others more. As your love increases, your FAITH and SELF -CONFIDENCE grows. As your F A I T H grows, your LOVE increases!

STOP THE READING! As you finish this portion, get your LAF NOTE-BOOK, and write down as many ways you can <u>LOVE and express love</u>, especially to and for yourself.

LOVE IS GIVING

As you start on this LOVE AWAY FAT MAP, you may, but not necessarily, feel vaguely uncomfortable or uneasy. As you continue, and as you LOVE YOURSELF MORE, these feelings will fade away and be replaced with feelings of confidence, self-assurance, and joy, even elation! Some of the steps and some of the positive affirmations may seem hypocritical at first. These too will vanish, being assured that you are embarking on a God-given way and a people-proven program. Any change in our lives, any different or unfamiliar way may bring feelings of uneasiness or awkwardness at first. LOVING YOURSELF MORE,
you persist right on through these.
(See TOGETHERNESS EXERCISE.)

You are not fooling yourself anymore. There is nothing fake about it. You are facing yourself squarely. You are building up a proper self-love which automatically moves you toward your better self, becoming your ideal size and weight, your God-intended self.

Dr. Cecil G. Osborne, in his book, "The Art Of Loving Yourself," states: "Both the alcoholic (and one might add drug addict, 'workaholic' and compulsive eater) and the one attempting to fake self-esteem, self-love are doomed to failure. The inner judge or conscience is not an enemy, but our friend. He is on our side, no matter how often we may fail. His ultimate goal is to help us avoid all actions or attitudes that prevent us from LOVING OURSELVES PROPERLY." (My emphasis.) You come to realize that LOVING YOURSELF MORE is not selfish or egotistical.

"If it is a virtue to love my neighbor as a human being, it must be a virtue —and not a sin —to love myself, since I am a human being too." Remember, Christ said, "Love your neighbor as yourself." Doesn't this indicate that we should already love ourselves?

Actually selfish people do not love themselves, they dislike themselves. In consultation with them, they sometimes actually use the words, "I hate myself." You learn to be aware of any such self-condemnation and change these negative self-criticizing and deprecating behaviors to self-accepting, loving and appreciating yourself more and more. You are ridding yourself of all such negative feelings about yourself, just as you would by dumping a load from your trouble wagon you have been pulling along behind you.

By Facing the situation, and determining how to better handle it in the future, you build "points" toward a better self-image, SELF-LOVE. You then have an inner force that helps you cope with future situations in a competent, self-assured manner.

LOVE is giving. So give to yourself. Give to yourself a clean bill of health. If you have been through more than the usual number of stressful events, within the last year particularly, have a complete physical check-up. Ask the doctor to check your blood sugar level. If you have had other unexplained symptoms_ lack of energy, head-aches, internal pain, etc., be sure to have your doctor to advise you. Be open. "Perfect LOVE cast out fear."[4]

So rather than continuing on along fearing that you have something drastically wrong, and not wanting to know about it, LOVE YOURSELF MORE by finding out for sure, and then doing whatever is necessary-if anything.

As you love yourself more, and accept the power of God's love within, your mind-brain transmits that changing power to every organ, gland and cell of your mind-brain-body. That wisdom knows what to do about the "fat cells," the "set points," the "metabolism," the "appetite" of your body.

Loving yourself more, your attitude changes, your behavior changes, your body chemicals and mechanism change and your habits all change for the better. Your appetite is for food only when your physical body in general is hungry and more specifically when your stomach is hungry. You now realize that hunger is that physiological lack.

You eat only when hungry and that *sparingly and property.*

A good guide to follow is AT EACH MEAL, <u>EAT ONLY ENOUGH TO HOLD YOU OVER UNTIL THE NEXT MEAL- WHICH IS NOT VERY LONG!</u> Many people eat beyond this point, thus having to store the overage as fat!

The hunger and satiety center, of the mind-brain are now more efficient, quickly responding and turning down the appestat, so you are satisfied, yet never feel uncomfortably full and stuffed.

Study the chart on page 136.

Notice a friend or an acquaintance who has a very nice figure - slim and trim. Compliment her on her figure; then ask her some questions about how she does it.
"Have you always been that way?" "Do you count calories?" etc. Have a meal together, and observe what and how much she eats.

THEN DEVELOP THE HABIT OF WATCHING YOURSELF; WHAT AND HOW MUCH **YOU** EAT.

In the meantime, you feel emotionally and spiritually satiated. Also you find that you automatically change self-defeating thoughts and feelings into positive self-achieving success thoughts and behavior.

As you read your LOVE AWAY FAT MAP, you learn to set realistic goals. Give yourself worthwhile goals. You can't swallow a whole apple in just one bite without choking on it, but with one bite at a time, it becomes delicious. So set realistic goals for yourself, rather than neurotic fantasies. Divide them into small bites that you can meet more and more easily. Achieve small successes at first, and then you will be in better position to set a more ambitious goal.

REFER TO GOAL SETTING, MY ACTIVATING PURPOSE, AND GOAL CARD 10..

A very important fact to face is that you can probably look great very attractive weighing a little more than you have thought about as your desired weight!
Be realistic in setting your goal-image weight, not necessarily as you were at sixteen, or when you married, or as your favorite movie star!

One problem many weight losers may have is that they want that new figure NOW! Maybe they are going to a big party next month, and they want to get into those clothes that have been hanging in the closet three years or more. LOVING YOURSELF MORE, practice patience along with determination and perseverance.

You are not a "weight loser;" YOU are a weight controller! And you more and more easily
LOVE AWAY UNWANTED POUNDS.
As you LOVE YOURSELF in a proper manner, you face your real self as you truly are.

You realize that you have many fine qualities. After reading LAF MAP all the way through, use your LAF NOTE BOOK, and make a list of your special attributes. Keep this private. Just God and you need to know about this. Thus you can feel free. List the traits you like, your character values, your achievements, any honors obtained, no matter how large or small. Also list what you like about your features, your eyes, lips, your hands, etc.

Now consider closely your INNER NEEDS *AND* **VALUES. What** is in this for you? Why do you want to change? What are your true BASIC ROOT NEEDS? Review: BASIC HUMAN NEEDS. Now stop reading and write these out. What are the REWARDS AND BENEFITS? Have you written them down? Each time you read them, and, when you come to this part, stop again; look at your rewards and benefits.. Add to these if you wish, Then continue.
You are not playing games with me or yourself, or anyone else. You are moving right to the basic, the root cause. You are stripping it of its compulsive power.

75

You are replacing it with the most powerful force of all, proper LOVE. You realize this is not a temporary program, like going on a diet or following the "xyz" plan. This *LOVING AWAY FAT way is a happy way of life, for life.* This is a universal way, which achieves for anyone..

Jesus said, "Give, and it will be given to you; good measure, pressed down, shaken together, running over, will be put into your lap. For the measure you give will be the measure you get back." You can't out-give God! Therefore LOVING YOURSELF MORE, GIVE LOVE, and you get LOVE. Starting with yourself give LOVE, care, acceptance, understanding, responsibility, forgiveness, and especially *FORGIVENESS.* As you give these and other LOVE-ACTIONS, you FEEL LOVED.

LOVING YOURSELF MORE, you are developing an inner attitude of giving.

LOVE is ACTION doing, giving of yourself. The following of this LOVE AWAY FAT MAP leads you to get to the root cause of your concerns, uproot them and plant a new LOVE, a new SELF-IMAGE. This self-love fulfills you mentally, physically and emotionally.

To help you to LOVE YOURSELF MORE, to have more acceptance, understanding, forgiveness, decide now that you will practice giving to others, not just accepting others only, but also giving praise, giving compliments.

As you look for ways to add good feelings, joy and happiness in other's lives, you find that you have good feelings, joy and happiness in your own life.

If at first you feel a little uncomfortable or have any other negative feelings in giving praise, just act as if it is the natural thing to do. We find that this sometimes works wonders. As you "act as if," soon you find you are no longer acting, and truly experience the real thing.

LOVING YOURSELF MORE, you are a giving person. Give of your time, sharing yourself with those who really need love, direction, care, a listening ear.

Many times people eat when they feel lonely or depressed, whether they are actually hungry or not. One of the effective ways to overcome these feelings, and at the same time fulfill (Fill Full) a lack in your life, is to share yourself with another, someone who has a need. LOVE follows action! Action follows LOVE! Write a letter, make a phone call, whatever, and put LOVE IN ACTION. Refer to "LOVE IN ACTION GROUP.".

(Author's note: Some of these suggestions are repeated to give a greater "hypnotic" benefit .)

LOVING YOURSELF MORE, you give *forgiveness.* First give it to yourself: After you have faced your *"goof,"* admitted it to God, <u>accept </u>His forgiveness. What do you still feel guilty about? Have you let some guilt go on over a period of time? That is not scriptural. "Ask and you shall receive. Perhaps you have confessed but have not appropriated existential forgiveness. Take the "and it so" attitude. "AMEN." "It is finished." This is the other side of forgiveness. "God is faithful and just and will forgive." What about you? Are you forgiving of yourself? Many people have a problem here. Punishment in many forms is brought upon them, not by God, not by others, but themselves, their own subconscious minds.

They have not relieved themselves of guilt through the worship of confession and the receiving of forgiveness. Read carefully the Guilt and Self-punishment section.

You are becoming keenly aware and very attentive to yourself, aware of your real needs. You give of yourself to yourself. You are kind, tenderhearted and forgiving. Now I want you to take time to write in your LAF NOTE BOOK answers to this question: "In what ways have I offended myself, ME?" IF any have not been confessed before, just point them out to God. He forgives you. I forgive you!

Make sure you forgive yourself. Write across each one "FORGIVEN!" Then repeat your love phrase: "LOVING MYSELF MORE, I am forgiven. I'm Free! I'm Free of any guilt! I don't owe anything." "Owe no one anything, except to love one another." "One", that's YOU. "Another," that's others. See Romans 13:6.

You LOVE YOURSELF MORE by giving in another way. You give to yourself the freedom of making mistakes. No one is perfect. IF you never do anything, you make no mistakes! Reading LAF, you will learn to look on mistakes as learning experiences. As you realize this more deeply, you find that you make fewer and fewer mistakes! You are admitting that it is OK to say: "I goofed," "1 was wrong," "forgive me." Saying "I'm sorry" is not as effective and healing as saying, "I was wrong, will you forgive me?" You are building yourself up rather than diminishing yourself by willingly admitting "I was wrong."

When you have appropriated forgiveness for yourself, you are in position to give forgiveness to others.

Give it even if those involved do not seek or ask forgiveness. Some people are vindictive, mean, cruel, wounding-sometimes intentional, and sometimes unintentional. Jesus said of his persecutors, "Forgive them, for they know not what they do."

To help you rid yourself of any remaining negative feelings .hurts, resentments, bitterness, anger, guilt .any and all, let this "Melting Away exercise" work for you.

MELT-AWAY-PROGRAM

You wake up to a bright sunny winter day. During the night a snow fell, leaving everything outside covered in a beautiful glistening blanket of white. The clouds have moved on. The temperature in the sunshine is mild, just right for making a snowman! You start rolling up a snowball for your snowman; only this one is done differently from any other. As you roll up more and more snow, you roll in those hurts, those feelings of anger, resentment, bitterness, guilt, any other negative destructive emotions that have bothered you in the least. Keep rolling them in until you have every one inside the snowball. Now take the snowball into the shower in the bathroom (you may need help!). Turn on the hot water and watch the snowball melt. Watch the water from the melted snow, mingled with the shower water and all the hurts, anger, resentment, bitterness along with the guilt, disappear down the drain, NEVER to be seen again! They are gone, and can never be put together again. They are gone from your life forever!

Another LOVE YOURSELF MORE gift that you can make sure you are giving to yourself is the "right" to change. You are free to change. You are free to right wrongs, not only within yourself but with those who would diminish you. When you let someone diminish you in whatever way, you are also letting that person subtract from himself.

To be fair, and to give love to others, and to yourself, you avoid letting others tear you down. You stand firm, remembering that LOVE IS THE CHANGING POWER. You have LOVE. You have POWER. Without anger, quietly, gently, but firmly and politely, you insist on people putting things right.

A LOVE IN ACTION way to build your SELF-LOVE - your SELF-ESTEEM is to give of yourself in active listening. We can get so involved in our own concerns that we may forget to hear. Give a hearing ear, hearing with your heart. You become aware of what the other person is really saying, and perhaps more importantly, really feeling. You listen for feelings.

You become genuinely interested in what that person has to say. You are more and more aware of others' true feelings. You respond to the feelings and listen. Respond to the feelings and listen. Respond to the feelings and --listen some more!
LOVING YOURSELF MORE, you give yourself the risk of rejection. Every salesperson has to risk rejection. But he knows that for every so many "no's", there is the big "yes", the acceptance. He knows it is worth all the "no's." Actually everyone is a salesperson in that they sell their ideas and personalities, etc., either positively or negatively. LOVE yourself, take that risk. Move on out, so you won't miss out on all the abundant living waiting for you.

Fear can say to you, "I may be rejected," "I may become embarrassed," "I don't want to look bad or say the wrong thing." So what! Watch the TV bloopers and you will realize a mistake is not the end! Launch out into the deep where you can enjoy life freely.

LOVING YOURSELF MORE, you give of yourself to others in a group. To build up SELF-LOVE, to prevent depression arid loneliness and feeling sorry for yourself, get with others. Get with a LOVE IN ACTION group, a synergistic group where people are interested in others, giving of themselves to each other and to special projects of helping people. The tasks may be simple, but you feel good, knowing that you are putting LOVE IN ACTION.

IF you are not presently in such a group, join one or form one. It is good to give and share with another one person, but also beneficial to join in with a group, preferably not too large a group. STOP READING. IF you are not in such a group, who and where can you join such a group? Write it down now. DECIDE.

LOVING YOURSELF MORE, you are kind to yourself. Give to yourself a Relaxation Retreat. At times it is good to withdraw temporarily; then after gathering strength charge ahead! Adjust and go ahead. It is good to have a place all to yourself--a place away from the busyness of business and family activities — a place where you can retreat, relax, rest, refresh and rejuvenate! Refer to: RELAXATION AND REJUVENATION SESSION, with the TOGETHERNESS EXERCISE,

Remember, Jesus laid it before us:
LOVE, LOVE, LOVE!

81

So LOVE IS THE CHANGING POWER:

LOVE of God from God, to God.

LOVE of others —to others, from others
LOVE of self —to self, from self,
ALL of your SELF, the adult-self and the
child-self.

Think **of all the ways you learned about the many forms in**
which LOVE has been manifested in your *life,* **comfort,**
caring. sympathy, and FOOD. Now That you are older, no
longer a small dependent child, you realize that food is
nutrition only. Your adult-self puts away from your
child-self the subconscious thoughts of relating food to love.
Your child-self feels cared for, sympathized with, comforted,
secure and loved, knowing that all needs are taken care of by
God through your adult-self. You feel pleased, happy,
safe and secure.

YOU LOVE YOURSELF.
YOU FEEL LOVED.

Let go of the past. You can't change the past, but you can
change the NOW and the FUTURE!
You realize the decisions you have made in the past have
brought you to your present condition. You can DECIDE -
PRE-DECIDE--NOW to change.

You also modify your thinking about exercise, realizing that
exercise alone cannot keep you at your goal-weight and
shape. You realize it can help tone you up, make you feel
better, look better and perk up your self-concept. You'll love
yourself more.

You also modify your eating behavior. The cues, the situations, the stimuli that in the past caused you to eat and/or overeat no longer entice you. You are FREE. No longer does TV and food go together, - nor do the TV commercials appeal to you at all. It's easier and easier to drive right on past the quick food drive-ins. Remember every time that you are tempted, that there many people out there who are succeeding in their weight reduction and control. You are one of them! Your inner mind (your subconscious) maintains a constant vigilance and the LIBERATING P O W E R O F LO V E c o m fo r t s y o u.

LOVE, ROMANCE, SEX AFFIRMATIONS

LOVING YOURSELF MORE, you now embark on ways to bring more ROMANCE into your life. Let the triune of LOVE, ROMANCE and SEX become complete in your life, then weight reduction follows naturally. You look for and find Things that bring interest, satisfaction, ROMANCE into your life! One can develop a love for one's work, avocation or a hobby.

As you have found out in Realization and Confession, many of your activities run counter to achieving your objective, and fulfilling your real basic needs; so now you are paying more attention to your activities. Become aware of any negative activities. Ask yourself, "If I love myself properly, will I continue in this activity?" The more LOVE, ROMANCE and SEX you can involve in these activities, the more effective they will be in moving you toward your goal image. I don't mean once a month or once a week. Why not every day?

With LOVING AWAY FAT, you find yourself modifying your attitude about food and how you use it.

You are becoming more and more aware of the misuse and thus find yourself changing that into a more satisfying behavior that brings pleasing results.

Even when your adult-self feels neglected in the triune of LOVE, ROMANCE and SEX, you are firm with your child-self and block any attempts of making food a substitute.

> FOOD is NOT LOVE.
> Food is not ROMANCE.
> Food is not SEX.
> Food is food and too much or
> the wrong kind for you causes problems.

LOVING YOURSELF MORE, look for ways to bring more interest, more romance into your work, your social life, your family life. You are to develop a dynamic, active attitude toward LOVE. Refuse to follow the herd of those inactive TV lovers and have an active pursuit of ROMANCE. Put ROMANCE into your life.

A person who has his or her "antenna" up, who is mentally and emotionally ready to receive love, and has the desire "tuned in" for the triune of LOVE, ROMANCE and SEX relationship, will find it drawn to him or her. Start on your adventure of ROMANCE. Start putting up your antenna NOW --TODAY. Pre-decide. Make the decision NOW that you ARE ROMANTIC.

> YOU LOVE YOURSELF.
> YOU FEEL LOVED.

> SAY IT **NOW;**
> I LOVE MYRSELF!.
> I FEEL LOVED!

With the LOVE AWAY FAT Way, you have
a way-of-life, not just a temporary program,
a diet, or technique or exercise. You have a
SATISFYING,   GRATIFYING,
WONDERFUL   WAY-OF-LIFE.

Loving yourself more, you accept yourself as you are
NOW.. .no matter what you feel or how
You look.

Then you find that you move forward to being loving, lovable and lovely (handsome)!

GOD DID NOT GIVE US
A SPIRIT OF TIMIDITY
BUT A SPIRIT OF POWER
AND
LOVE AND SELF CONTROL.

II Timothy 1:7 RSV.

DO I LOVE YOU?
God knows I do!   Joe
2 Corinthians 11:11

BIBLIOGRAPHY-RESOURCES

INTRODUCTION/EXPLANATION

1. EUGENE SCHEIMANN, <u>Sex and The Over-Weight Woman</u>.
2.   (New York: Signet Books, l97O)pl5
2. Leo Buscaglio, LOVE..(New York: Fawcett Crest, l978),p7l

ROOT CAUSE

1. RICHARD MASHBUIRN, <u>Eat and Grow SIim</u>,.p23
2. Johann Wolfgang Von Goethe
3. Smiley Blanton, <u>Love or Perish</u>
4 ibid
5. Napoleon Hill, <u>Think and Grow Rich</u>(Cleveland, Ohio: The Ralston Co.),p[297]
6. Nathaniel Brandon, <u>The Psvchology of Self-Esteem</u>: (Bantam Books, Inc. 1969)
7. Norman Vincent Peale and Smiley Blanton, <u>Faith Is The Answer</u>
8. James Mallory, <u>The Kink and I</u>
9. I Corinthians 13
10. l John 4:18 RSV
11. Wayne Dyer, <u>Your Erroneous Zones</u>
12. Napoleon Hill, ibid
13. E. Stanley Jones, <u>Victory Through Surrender</u>
14. 1 John 4:8-10 RSV
15. Brian Tracy, <u>The Psychology of Achievement</u>

ANGER/GUILT/SELF-PUNISHMENT

1. Ephesians 4:31
2. Romans 12:I9 RSV.
3. Polston, <u>There Can Be a New You</u>
4. Mathew:I4 RSV

FOOD—SECURITY—LOVE

1. Genesis 1:27 RSV
2. 1 John 4:16
3. John 14:15, Mathew22:37RSV
4. Psalms *8:5* RSV
5. John 13:34
6. Luke 6:38
7. Matthew 22:39
8. Eric Fromm, The Art of Lovin2
9. 1 John 4:18
10. Theodore J. Smith, American Institute of Hvonosis Journal
11. Muriel James, Born To Live
12. Theodore J. Smith, ibid

YOUR SECURITY GUARD

Nathaniel Brandon, The Psycholoay of Self-Esteem, New York: Bantam Books,Inc.'69.

COMPULSIVE EATING

1. Eugene Scheimann, Sex and The Overweight Woman

LOVE, ROMANCE, SEX

1. ibid
2. Albert Schweitzer
3. Eugene Schliemann, ibid

OTHER PEPS and PIMS

1. 1 John 4:18
2. Psalms 103: 12
3. 1John l:9
4. Ephesians 2:4
5. II Peter3:9
6. Mathew 5:24

LOVE IS THE CHANGING POWER

1. Proverbs 23:7 KJV.

HOW CAN YOU HELP YOURSELF

1. Cecil Osborne, You're In Charge. New York: Pillar Books, 1973 p20
2. Dale Galloway, How To Feel Like a---
3. Mildred Newman and Bernard Berkowitz. How to Be Your Own Best Friend
4. Leo Buscaglia, Living, Loving, Learning
5. I Johni:9
6. John 8:36

POSI-PEP/PUNISHMENT

1. I Corinthians 14:1

IDENTIFICATION

1. E. Stanley Jones, ibid
2. 1 Corinthians 14:20 NED, RSV
3. I Corinthians 14:1

LOVE IS GIVING

1. Cecil Osborne, The Art of Loving Yourself p100
2. Eric Fromm, Art Of Loving.
   (N.Y.: Harper and Row, 1956 p56)
3. Luke 10:27
4. 1John 4:18
5. Luke6:38,NEB

Also see: David Dunn, Try Giving Yourself Away; Carmel, N.Y.

Guideposts Associates, Inc.)

Og Mandino, The Greatest Salesman In The World (New York: Frederick Fell, Inc.)

See especially The Scroll Marked II.

LOVE IS ACTION

1. Mathew 7:7KJV
2. 1John l:9 KJV   3.   Luke 23:34

(For your LAF NOTE BOOK)

_MY_ SPECIAL ATTRIBUTES

List here my special attributes. Keep this private. Just God and I need to know about this. Thus I can feel free to let go. List the traits I like, the character values, my personality. my achievements, any honors obtained. What I like about my features-- — my eyes, lips, hands, etc.

GOAL SETTING,
MAP-My Activating Purpose

Loving yourself more, you are to set goals that are consistent with what you can conceive and believe. What do you _really_ **WANT-DESIRE DEEPLY?** The very act of writing these down is giving a powerful AFFIRMATION, a strong influence, and a potent control to your inner mind to do something about them. Thus you are WRITING YOUR **SCRIPT** FOR NOW AND THE FUTURE   You are determining in your **_body, mind and spirit_** EXACTLY what you want to be, what you are ready to be.

Loving yourself ENOUGH, you make a commitment.

You DECIDE NOW once and for all.

SCRIPT. CARD: MY GOAL

I do concentrate on this:

I LEAVE the past behind and

with hands outstretched to whatever lies ahead

I go straight for the goal - my reward the honor

of my high calling by God in Christ Jesus."

Philippians 3:13&14 (Phillips)

Loving yourself more, you set "check-up" times and follow through.

GOAL CARD 10

Loving myself more, by_____(Mo., Day, year)
I am going to weigh_____pounds.
I am going to be size____in waist and (list places important to you.)
This means I am going to remove an average of
___excess pounds per week.

My LOVE increases as my WEIGHT decreases!

The "END"— the BOTTOM LINE the ULTIMATE GOAL is

LOVE .
1. out of a pure heart

2. of a good conscience

3. of unfeigned Faith.

(See I Timothy 1:5 KJV.)

(For your LAF NOTE BOOK)

REWARDS AND BENEFITS

WHAT **are the <u>REWARDS and BENEFITS </u>for ME?**
What's in it for ME? Remember this is not selfish; it is
loving **yourself more, and thus you can** love **others more!**

Some of these BENEFITS may be antonyms to the
negatives written before.

A NEED or LACK fulfilled is a BENEFIT and a REWARD! This
becomes your new
POSI-PEP/POSI-PIM.

"FAILURE TO
PROPERLY LOVE
MYSELF CAUSES
ME T0 BE UNABLE
T0 PROPERLY
LOVE OTHERS"

LOVE CARD

On a 3x5 card list ways to LOVE --GIVE. God so LOVED that he GAVE. God is LOVE. LOVE is GIVING.
Pick one category EACH DAY and emphasize that one, continuing to GIVE of other categories as opportunities present themselves.
For God so LOVED the world that he GAVE his only son, that whoever believes in him should not perish but hove eternal life .[1]
Everyone who believes that Jesus is the Christ is a child of God, and everyone who LOVES the parent LOVES the child.[2] **By** this we know LOVE, that he laid down [GAVE] his life for us. .[3]
See what LOVE the Father has GIVEN us, that we should be called children of God.
God is LOVE, and he who abides in LOVE abides in God, and God abides in him.[5]
We LOVE because he First LOVED us.[6]
Little children, let us not LOVE merely in theory or in wards,-— let us LOVE in sincerity and in practice![7]

LOVE CARD
* GRATITUDE— THANKS
* TIME
• ENERGY
• ACCEPTANCE
• APPROVAL
* AFFIRMATION
* FRIENDSHIP GOODWILL
• FORGIVENESS
  TOUCHING IN PERSON
      BY LETTER
• BY PHONE &
• COMPLIMENTS
• ABCs of GOOD NEWS

GIVE LOVE
    IN WHAT WAYS CAN I LOVE AND EXPRESS LOVE?
HOW TO USE THE LAF and SCRIPT CARDS

Any way that you use the LAF and SCRIPT CARDS will probably be effective. However by following these simple steps, the effectiveness can be multiplied many times.

Choose a LAF CARD and/or SCRIPT CARD that has special meaning for you. COPY and carry with you. A 3x5 inch card is a good size. The SCRIPT CARDS have a double impact:
1. **Scriptural**, and 2. A powerful inspiring **SCRIPT** FOR YOUR role in life; you act out that script.
2. <u>**The SCRIPT. CARD'S scripture is personalized**</u>.

First use the Togetherness Exercise, thus preparing your mind-brain, causing it to be more receptive and responsive to the card affirmations.

MAKE MENTAL MOVIES ~

This is the LOVE-VISION technique which is hypnotic in effect. With this procedure, you get the proper message to the place in your mind-brain where behavior is affected. It helps you to recondition and re-educate your INNER MIND, Thus you are *rewriting* your SCRIPT. And you are going to act out that new and better script!

Holding the LAF CARD or SCRIPT. CARD before you, let your creative mind take over.   Realize in your imagination, you can he anywhere, anytime, with anyone. So as you look at the LAF CARD or SCRIPT. CARD; couple your imagination with your Feelings, and SEE AND FEEL AND BELIEVE THE AFFIRMATION.

Go over the affirmation slowly, thoughtfully and meditatively SEVEN TIMES.

100

LAF CARD 1

WITH THE
LOVE AWAY FAT M.A.P,

I HAVE PERMANENT SUCCESS!

....

LAF CARD 2

IT IS EASY AS I BUILD LOVE
AND CONFIDENCE

FOLLOWING THE LOVE AWAY FAT M.A.P

....

LAF CARD 3

LOVE IS THE GREATEST MOVING FORCE

6

....

100

LAF CARD 4

BY READING THE LAF AFFIRMATIONS
REGULARLY, I RID MYSELF
OF SELF-DEFEATING BEHAVIOR

....

LAF CARD 5

I AM MAKING SURE THAT I HAVE
THE RIGHT PEPs AND PIMs OPERATING WITHIN.

....

LAF CARD 6

I HAVE THE JOY AND HAPPINESS
OF A LOVING ADULT.

LAF CARD ~7

I CAN BE WHAT I WANT TO BE AS A RESULT

OF   "THE LOVING MYSELF" MORE" WAY.

....

LAF CARD 8

I REALIZE THAT LOVE 1S THE CHANGING POWER.

I AM A LOVING PERSON. I LOVE MYSELF.

I AM DOING GOOD THINGS FOR MYSELF.

I AM KIND TO MYSELF AND DO KIND THINGS

FOR MYSELF AS WELL AS OTHERS.

....

LAF CARD 9

AS I LOVE MYSELF MORE,
MY FAITH IS BECOMING STRONGER.
I AM MORE SELF CONFIDENT AND
SELF-ASSURED.

....

GOAL CARD. M.A.P.

My Activating PURPOSE

I READ MY GOAL CARD AT LEAST

TWICE DAILY- WHEN I AWAKEN AND

BEFORE I GO TO SLEEP

....

GOAL CARD 10

I am going to weigh_____pounds by
_____(Mo.,Day,Year), removing an average of____
excess pounds per week. My waist is goingto be____.
In LOVING MYSELF MORE, I GIVE to myself an ACTIVE
ATTITUDE OF AWARENESS. Thus I eat SLOWLY,
SPARINGLY and SIMPLY —TODAY AND EVERYDAY.
"SPARINGLY" is the right amounts, and "SIMPLY" is the
RIGHT KIND OF FOOD ONLY, and at the RIGHT TIMES
and PLACES. My LOVE is increasing, and as my LOVE
increases, my FAITH and SELF   CONFIDENCE increase.
I SEE IT, I FEEL IT,
        I BELIEVE IT!   AND IT IS SO!
....

.

LAF CARD 11.

VISUALIZE MY SIZE!

....

LAF CARD 12

BE WISE,
VISUALIZE,
EXERCISE, AND
REALIZE !

....

LAF CARD 13

IMAGINE THE GOAL

PLAY THE ROLE
and

I HAVE CONTROL !

....

LAF CARD 14

I AM DEVELOPING A DYNAMIC ACTIVE
ATTITUDE TOWARD L.R.S., ESPECIALLY LOVE.

....

LAF CARD 15

LOVE IS THE CHANGING POWER.

GOD'S LOVE HELPS ME TO

FORGIVE FULLY, FREELY AND FINALLY.

....

LAF CARD 16

LOVING MYSELF MORE, I LOOK FOR WAYS
TO BRING MORE INTEREST, MORE ROMANCE
INTO MY WORK, MY SOCIAL LIFE
AND MY HOME LIFE.

.... LAF

CARD 17

I AM PREPARED FOR ALL KINDS
OF NEGATIVE SITUATIONS.

I AM FORTIFIED FROM WITHIN,
SECURE IN MY DEEP INNER
LOVE FOR MYSELF.

....

.

LAF CARD 18

INFINITE LOVE ENVELOPS ME,
HOLDS ME, COMFORTS ME,
PROTECTS ME,
AND SECURES ME.

I FEEL CONTENTED AND SATISFIED.

....

LAF CARD 19

LOVE HAS CREATED
AN INVISIBLE SHIELD ABOUT ME.

THOUGHTS OPPOSED TO MY GOAL-IMAGE
CANNOT PENETRATE THIS SHIELD OF LOVE.
I FEEL SAFE SECURE AND SERENE.

....

LAF CARD 20
MY LOVE FOR MYSELF STRENGTHENS ME
IN MY ACCOUNTABILITY.
MY LOVE BEARS FRUIT OF
RESPONSIBILITY AND SELF CARE.

LAF CARD 21

I REALIZE THAT THE EMOTIONS ARE THE
GREATEST FORCES IN MY LIFE, AND
LOVE IS THE GREATEST EMOTION- SO
LOVE IS THE GREATEST FORCE.

LOVE IS THE CHANGING POWER.

LAF CARD 22

I AM KIND, **FORGIVING** AND ACCEPTING.

LAF CARD 23

IT IS THRILLING TO CHANGE. IT'S EXCITING!

I GET MORE SATISFACTION AND
PLEASURE FROM CHANGING.

LAF CARD 2ᵗ4

WHEN I AM ALONE, WHEN MY FAMILY IS GONE,
I STILL FEEL SELF-ASSURED,
SELF-SUFFICIENT AND LOVED.

I FEEL SECURE.   I DO GOOD THINGS FOR MYSELF.

....

LAF CARD 25

I All INDEPENDENT..
I STAND ON MY OWN FEET.

....
LAF CARD 26

I AM MOVING AWAY FROM THE SO-CALLED
SATISFYING BEHAVIOR OF THE PAST WITH
UNSATISFACTORY RESULTS.

I AM MOVING TO PLEASING BEHAVIOR
NOW AND IN THE FUTURE, THUS
LEADING ME TO SATISFYING BENEFITS-
A SELF-LOVING, APPRECIATING SELF-IMAGE.

....

LAF CARD 27

LOVE IS ASSUMING RESPONSIBILITY
FOR SELF.

LOVING MYSELF MORE,
I ASSUME THAT RESPONSIBILITY..

....

LAF CARD 28

LOVING MYSELF MORE, I AM AWARE OF
WHAT, WHEN AND WHERE MY BEHAVIOR DOES
NOT HELP ME ACHIEVE THE GOAL IMAGE
I TRULY DESIRE.

....

LAF CARD 29

LOVING MYSELF MORE, I AM LETTING GO
OF PAST DEBILITATING BEHAVIOR..

I AM WELCOMING THE CHANGE
COMING INTO MY LIFE.

I'M FREE TO CHANGE!

....

LAF CARD 30

I AM LOOKING FORWARD WITH
PLEASURABLE ANTICIPATION TO
CHANGING INTO **A BETTER ME**!

....

LAF CARD 31

LOVING MYSELF MORE,
I <u>LET GO</u> OF ANY <u>ANGER</u>.
I AM FREE TO TURN
AWAY.

I AM FREE TO **<u>LET GO</u>**!

....

LAF CARD 32

I AM "DUMPING" ANY RESENTMENT,
ANY BITTERNESS, ANY GRIEVANCE,
AND ANY REVENGEFUL ATTITUDE..
<u>I AM FREE</u> OF THAT <u>HEAVY LOAD</u>

....

LAF CARD 33

LOVING MYSELF MORE,
I AM FREE TO HAVE A
HIGH, HAPPY AND HEALTHY LIFE.

....

LAF CARD 34

I AM CLOSING THE DOOR BEHIND
TO THE FEAR OF DISAPPROVAL,
FEAR OF FAILURE,
PEAR OF HURTING,
AND FEAR OF DEFEAT..

LAF CARD 35

I All DEVELOPING MORE PATIENCE,
MORE PERSEVERANCE,
MORE DETERMINATION.

....

LAF CARD 36

LOVING MYSELF MORE,
I PRACTICE PATIENCE,
ALONG WITH DETERMINATION
AND PERSEVERANCE,

....

LAF CARD 37

I FEEL SELF-ASSURED..

I HAVE MORE COURAGE AND

MORE AND MORE CONFIDENCE.

....

LAF CARD 38

I VISUALIZE MYSELF AS I WANT TO BE..

I AM BECOMING WHAT I WANT TO BE.

....

LAF CARD 39

I AM SELF-ASSURED, SELF-SUFFICIENT AND
SELF-LOVED.   THUS I CAN SHARE
MORE LOVE WITH OTHERS AROUND ME.

....

LAF CARD   40

IT BECOMES EASY AND AUTOMATIC
TO FOLLOW A SELF-LOVING MODE OF LIVING,
TAKING NOTHING INTO MY BODY TO
MAR OR SCAR IT OR TO LOAD IT DOWN.

....

LAF CARD 41

I AM TAKING CHARGE. I AM TAKING HOLD
OF MYSELF AS A LOVING PARENT
TAKES CHARGE OF A MISBEHAVING CHILD.
THE CHILD-SELF UNDERSTANDS **A FIRM NO**.

....

LAF CARD 42₂

"DO NOT BE CHILDREN IN YOUR THINKING,
BUT IN THINKING; BE MATURE."
I COR. 14:20

....

CARD 43

I AM A UNIQUE PERSON.
. I AM CONFIDENT..
I HAVE A QUIET DETERMINATION
TO SURPASS MY PREVIOUS ACHIEVEMENTS.

....

LAF CARD 44

LOVING MYSELF MORE, I PUT INTO
ACTION WAYS TO BRING MORE
LOVE, ROMANCE AND SEX INTO MY LIFE

....

LAF CARD 45

THE WISDOM AND POWER WITHIN
GUIDES ME IN HANDLING ANGER
IN A LOVING CONSTRUCTIVE WAY.

....

LAF CARD 46

I ACT ON MY LOVE.
I RESOLVE TO USE FOOD ONLY FOR NUTRITION,
AND SINCE IT IS FOR NUTRITION ONLY,
I EAT SLOWLY, SPARINGLY AND SIMPLY,
AND IT IS SO!

....

LAF CARD 47

I DO MY EXERCISES RELIGIOUSLY.

I LOVE AWAY FAT WITH EXERCISES,
AND GOOD NUTRITION.

I IMPROVE MY OVERALL FITNESS

....

LAF CARD 48

I SOCIALIZE WHILE I EXERCISE.

WITH A FRIEND,
EXERCISE IS FUN!

.... LAF

CARD 49

LOVING MYSELF MORE,
I EXERCISE TO H E L P
REACH AND MAINTAIN
MY IDEAL WEIGHT AND SIZE.

....

LAF CARD 50,
"I WILL GREET THIS DAY WITH LOVE IN MY HEART.

And most of all I will love myself. For when I do I will zealously
inspect all things which enter my body, my mind,   my soul, and my heart. Never will I overindulge the requests of my flesh; rather I will cherish my body with cleanliness and moderation. Never will I allow my mind to be attracted to evil and despair; rather I will uplift it with the knowledge and wisdom of the ages. Never will I allow my soul to become complacent and satisfied, rather I will feed it with meditation and prayer. Never will I allow my heart to become small and bitter, rather I will share it and
it will grow and warm the earth."

From "The Greatest Salesman In The World",
By Og Mondino.

ADDITIONAL LAF TEXT FOR CARDS

I AM PUTTING MORE LOVE, ROMANCE AND
SEX INTO MY LIFE.

LOVING MYSELF MORE, I PUT INTO ACTION
WAYS TO BRING MORE LOVE, ROMANCE AND
SEX INTO MY LIFE..

I AM MORE AND MORE MENTALLY AND
EMOTIONAL READY TO RECEIVE LOVE.
.. I HAVE MY DESIRE TUNED IN FOR
THE TRIUNE OF LOVE. ROMANCE AND
SEX RELATIONSHIP.
THUS I FIND IT DRAWN TO ME!

I AM LETTING THE TRIUNE OF LOVE, ROMANCE
AND SEX BECOME COMPLETE IN MY I.IFE.

THE MORE L.R.S. I INVOLVE IN MY ACTIVITIES,
THE MORE EFFECTIVE THEY BECOME IN
MOVING ME TO MY GOAL **IMAGE**.

I AM DEVELOPING A DYNAMIC ACTIVE
ATTITUDE TOWARD L.R.S., ESPECIALLY LOVE.

I REFUSE TO FOLLOW THE HERD OF THOSE
INACI'IVE TV LOVERS AND BEGIN PURSUING
LOVE, ROMANCE AND SEX!

....

SCRIPT. CARD 51.

WHETHER I EAT OR DRINK, OR

WHATEVER I AM DOING, I DO ALL

FOR THE HONOR OF GOD.

1 COR.10:31 NEB. PERSONALIZED

··

SCRIPT.. CARD 52

I KNOW THAT MY BODY IS A TEMPLE OF

THE HOLY SPIRIT WITHIN ME, WHICH I HAVE

FROM GOD. SO I GLORIFY GOD IN MY BODY.

1 COR. 6:19 RSV PERSONALIZED

.

··

SCRIPT. CARD 53

IN ALL THESE THINGS,
I AM MORE THAN CONQUEROR
THROUGH HIM WHO LOVES ME

.ROMANS 8:37 RSV. PERSONALIZED

··

SCRIPT. CARD 54

FOR THE MOMENT ALL DISCIPLINE SEEMS
PAINFUL RATHER THAN PLEASANT;
LATER IT YIELDS THE PEACEFUL
FRUIT OF RIGHTEOUSNESS TO ME
WHEN I HAVE BEEN TRAINED BY IT.
HEBREWS 12:11 RSV.

··

SCRIPT. CARD 55

I HAVE NO ROOM FOR FEAR IN LOVE;
PERFECT LOVE BANISHES FEAR.

1 JOHN 4:19 NEB.

··
··

SCRIPT. CARD 56

LET ME GO ON LOVING OTHERS;
FOR LOVE COMES FROM GOD.
GOD IS LOVE; AS I DWELL IN LOVE,
I AM DWELLING IN GOD, AND GOD IN ME.
1JOHN 4:7 PHILLIPS & 8 NEB

··

SCRIPT. CARD 57

I DO NOT LOVE THE WORLD
OR THE
THINGS IN THE WORLD.
I AM KEEPING MYSELF IN
THE LOVE OF GOD!
1 JOHN 2: 15 and JUDE 21 RSV.

··

SCRIPT. CARD 58

ABOVE ALL, I AM KEEPING MY LOVE

FOR MYSELF AND OTHERS AT FULL STRENGTH,

BECAUSE LOVE CANCELS INNUMERABLE SINS.

1 PETER 4:8 NEB.

··

SCRIPT. CARD 59

IN LOVING MY MATE,
I LOVE MYSELF-MY BODY;
FOR I DO NOT HATE MY OWN FLESH,
BUT I NOURISH AND CHERISH IT
.
EPHESIANS 5:28&29 PERSONALIZED

....

SCRIPT. CARD 60

GOD DID NOT GIVE ME A SPIRIT OF

TIMIDITY, BUT A SPIRIT OF POWER

AND **LOVE** AND **SELF-CONTROL**.

2 TIMOTHY 1:7 RSV.. PERSONALIZED

....

SCRIPT. CARD 61

I DON'T LET THE WORLD AROUND ME
SQUEEZE ME INTO IT'S OWN MOLD, BUT
I LET GOD REMOLD MY MIND FROM WITHIN,
SO THAT I MAY PROVE IN PRACTICE THAT
THE PLAN OF GOD FOR ME IS GOOD,
MEETS ALL HIS DEMANDS AND MOVES ME
TOWARD THE GOAL OF TRUE MATURITY.

ROMANS 12:2 PHILLIPS PERSONAL I ZED

....

SCRIPT. CARD 62

AS I JUDGE NOT, I WILL NOT BE JUDGED; CONDEMN
NOT AND I WILL NOT BE CONDEMNED.
AS I FORGIVE, I WILL BE FORGIVEN.

LUKE 6:37 & 38 RSV.. PERSONALIZED

SCRIPT. CARD 63

I OWE NO ONE ANYTHING,
EXCEPT TO LOVE OTHERS AND
MYSELF PROPERLY;
FOR AS I LOVE OTHERS,
I HAVE FULFILLED THE LAW

ROMANS 13:6 RSV.. PERSONALIZED

SCRIPT. CARD 64

LOVING MORE, I AM PATIENT AND KIND
TO MYSELF AND TO OTHERS;
LOVING, I AM NOT JEALOUS
OR BOASTFUL.

I CORINTHIANS 13:4 RSV. PERSONALI ZED

SCRIPT. CARD 65

IN LOVING MYSELF AND OTHERS MORE,
I AM NOT CONCEITED NOR RUDE;
I AM NEVER SELFISH, NOR QUICK
TO TAKE OFFENCE. I KEEP
NO SCORE OF WRONGS, AND DO NOT GLOAT.
I DELIGHT IN THE TRUTH.

I CORINTHIANS 13:5&6 RSV.. PERSONALI ZE

....

SCRIPT. CARD 66

I MAKE LOVE MY AIM

I CORINTHIANS 14:1   RSV. PERSONALIZED

....

SCRIPT.. CARD 67

I AM NOT GOING TO BE CHILDISH

IN MY THINKING, BUT IN THINKING

I AM BEING MATURE

I CORINTHIANS 14:20 RSV. PERSONALIZED

....

SCRIPT. CARD 68

I HAVE CALMED AND QUIETED MY SOUL
PSALMS 131:2 RSV., PERSONALIZE

....

SCRIPT. CARD 69

I All LETTING THE LOVE OF CHRIST
CONTROL ME.

2 CORINTHIANS 5:14 RSV. PERSONALIZED

....

SCRIPT. CARD 70

Living by the Spirit's Power,
SO I SAY, I LET THE HOLY SPIRIT GUIDE MY LIFE.
THEN I WON'T BE DOING WHAT
MY SINFUL NATURE CRAVES.

GALATIANS 5:16   NLT   PERSONALIZED

....

SCRIPT. CARD 71

THE FRUIT OF THE SPIRIT IS
LOVE JOY, PEACE, PATIENCE, KINDNESS,
GOODNESS, FAITHFULNESS,
GENTLENESS, AND **SELF CONTROL**

GALATIANS 5: 22&23   RSV. PERSONALIZED

....
.

SCRIPT. CARD 72

NOW I PUT THEM ALL AWAY. ANGER,
WRATH, MALICE, SLANDER, AND FOUL
TALK. I PUT ON THEN, AS GOD'S CHOSEN
ONE, COMPASSION, KINDNESS, LOWLINESS,
MEEKNES9,AND **PATIENCE**-
COLOSSIANS 3:8&12 RSV. PERSONALIZED

....

SCRIPT. CARD 73

ABOVE, I PUT ON **LOVE**, WHICH BINDS

EVERYTHING TOGETHER IN PERFECT

HARMONY

COLOSSIANS 3:17 RSV. PERSONAL I ZED

....

SCRIPT. CARD 74

WHATEVER I DO, IN WORD OR DEED,

I DO EVERYTHING IN THE NAME

OF THE LORD JESUS, GIVING

THANKS TO GOD THE FATHER

THROUGH HIM.

COLOSSIANS 3:17 .PERSONAL I ZED

....

SCRIPT. CARD 75

I HAVE STRENGTH FOR ANYTHING

THROUGH HIM WHO GIVES ME POWER!

PHILIPPIANS 4:13 NEB. PERSONALIZED

....

SCRIPT. CARD 76

I SET MY AFFECTION ON THINGS ABOVE,

NOT ON THINGS ON THE EARTH

COLOSSIANS 3:2 KJV. PERSONALIZED

....

SCRIPT. CARD 77

MY ULTIMATE AIM, MY OBJECTIVE,
THE BOTTOM LINE IS **LOVE** WHICH
SPRINGS FROM A CLEAN HEART, FROM A
GOOD CONSCIENCE, AND FROM FAITH
THAT IS GENUINE.

I TIi1OTHY 1:5 NEB. PERSONALIZED

··

SCRIPT. CARD 78

THE POWER AT WORK WITHIN ME
IS ABLE TO DO FOR MORE ABUNDANTLY
THAN ALL I ASK OR THINK.

EPHESIANS 3:20 RSV..PERSONALIZED

··

SCRIPT. CARD 79

I WILL NOT GROW WEARY IN WELL DOING,

FOR IN DUE SEASON I SHALL REAP

BY NOT LOSING HEART!

GALATIANS 6:9 RSV. PERSONALIZED

SCRIPT. CARD 80

I AM STRENGTHENED WITH MIGHT
THROUGH HIS SPIRIT IN MY INNER BEING;
BEING **ROOTED AND GROUNDED IN LOVE.**

EPHESIANS 3:16,17 RSV. & NEB. PERSONALIZE

HURT MAP

DIRECTIONS FOR USE

Have you ever seen a highway map that wasn't cluttered? They look so confusing when you first pick them up! *Yet,* maps are made to help you to eliminate the confusion, keep you from getting lost and help you get to where you want to go in the best possible way. That is the purpose of HURT MAP. If maps are simplified too much they lose their usefulness. We want this map to be very useful and helpful.

I have in front of me a Rand McNally Interstate map of the United States.   First I look for my home town, Memphis, Tennessee.   Next I look for my goal destination, let's say Columbia, South Carolina for example. Now with my destination in sight, I begin to lose some of the cluttered feeling. By reading the highway signs and other directions, I can choose the route that I like, the one that best suits me. Do I want to go through Nashville and Knoxville and the mountains and have interstate highway all the way, or do I want to take U.S. 78 through Birmingham and Atlanta, and visit some friends and relatives along the way?   I have to **choose** which road. So it is with YOUR HURT MAP.

You must choose which road you will take. Then as you travel over the highways, you must continue to read the highway signs and markers. They're important! The numbers on the HURT MAP signs are references and have a corresponding reference "road sign" at the bottom of the map.

BE SURE TO STUDY THEM

Just as you would a new and strange highway map.

As you look at the map, do you find yourself in the highway of "RAGE" or "FURY," or did you bypass these but still find you are stuck with "resentment"? Have you followed the route of turning the negative feelings "OUTWARD"? Or do you have a tendency to turn them "INWARD" and "SEETHE"? Does the hurt you've endured make you boil inside? Have you recognized and faced the guilt that you carry along life's highway? If you feel guilty, why not dump it?

God does not want you to continue on with guilt. See more on guilt in "Handling Offenses", Also read the section on "Anger, Guilt and Self-Punishment,"

As you cross over to the better route, do you find that you can forgive others and ask forgiveness from God, but still find the huge obstacle of "SELF" blocking the way? Have you forgiven YOURSELF? Have you accepted God's forgiveness? Forgiveness from others?

Take your time. Don't speed. Read all the signs and all of the references. Then look at the "Fruits". Mark the ones that apply to you. Do you like what you see?

Do you need to make a turn- around or **cross over** to another route? Do you need to go by the "Pride Dump"?
Why settle for weeds when you could have "Fruits of The Good Harvest"?

HAVE A BEAUTIFUL AND REWARDING TRIP!

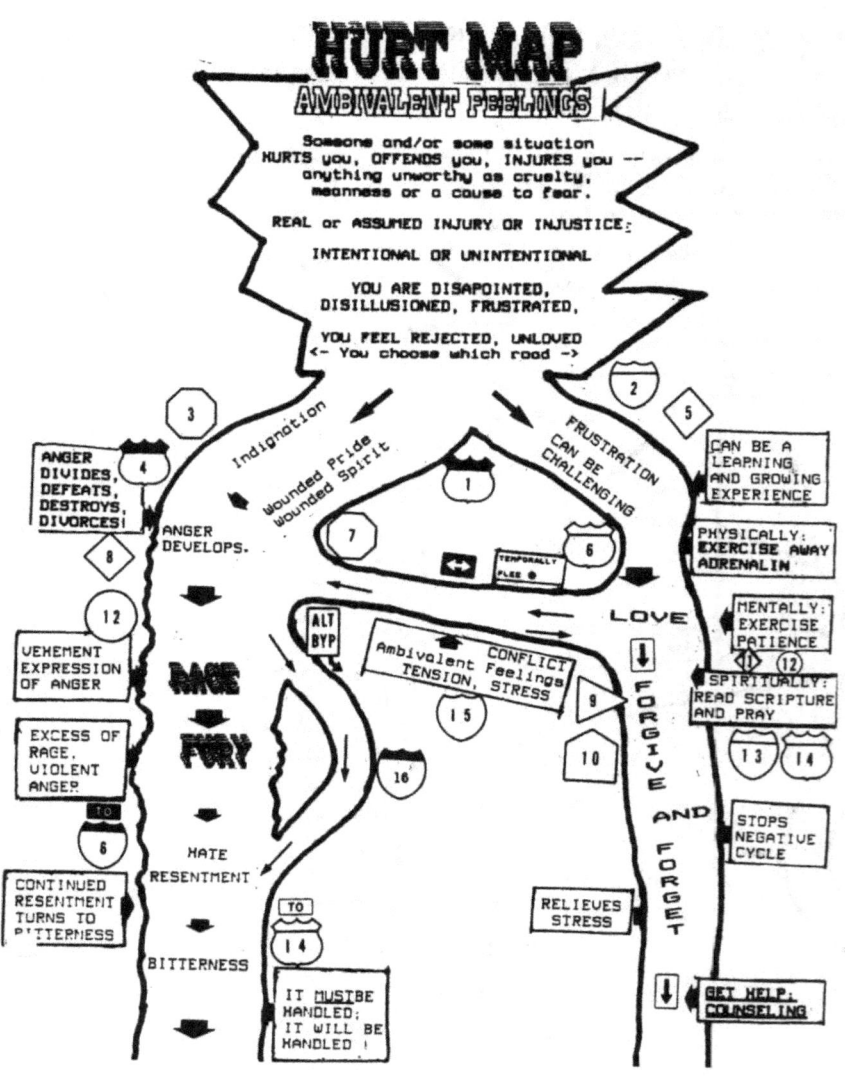

HURT MAP
AMBIVALENT FEELINGS

Someone and/or some situation
HURTS you, OFFENDS you, INJURES you --
anything unworthy as cruelty,
meanness or a cause to fear.

REAL or ASSUMED INJURY OR INJUSTICE:

INTENTIONAL OR UNINTENTIONAL

YOU ARE DISAPOINTED,
DISILLUSIONED, FRUSTRATED,

YOU FEEL REJECTED, UNLOVED
<- You choose which road ->

Indignation

Wounded Pride
wounded Spirit

FRUSTRATION
CAN BE
CHALLENGING

CAN BE A
LEARNING
AND GROWING
EXPERIENCE

PHYSICALLY:
EXERCISE AWAY
ADRENALIN

ANGER
DIVIDES,
DEFEATS,
DESTROYS,
DIVORCES!

ANGER
DEVELOPS.

TEMPORALLY
FLEE

MENTALLY:
EXERCISE
PATIENCE

LOVE

VEHEMENT
EXPRESSION
OF ANGER

RAGE

ALT
BYP

Ambivalent Feelings
TENSION, STRESS

CONFLICT

FORGIVE

SPIRITUALLY:
READ SCRIPTURE
AND PRAY

EXCESS OF
RAGE,
VIOLENT
ANGER.

FURY

AND

STOPS
NEGATIVE
CYCLE

TO

CONTINUED
RESENTMENT
TURNS TO
BITTERNESS

HATE
RESENTMENT

FORGET

RELIEVES
STRESS

BITTERNESS

TO

IT MUSTBE
HANDLED;
IT WILL BE
HANDLED !

GET HELP;
COUNSELING

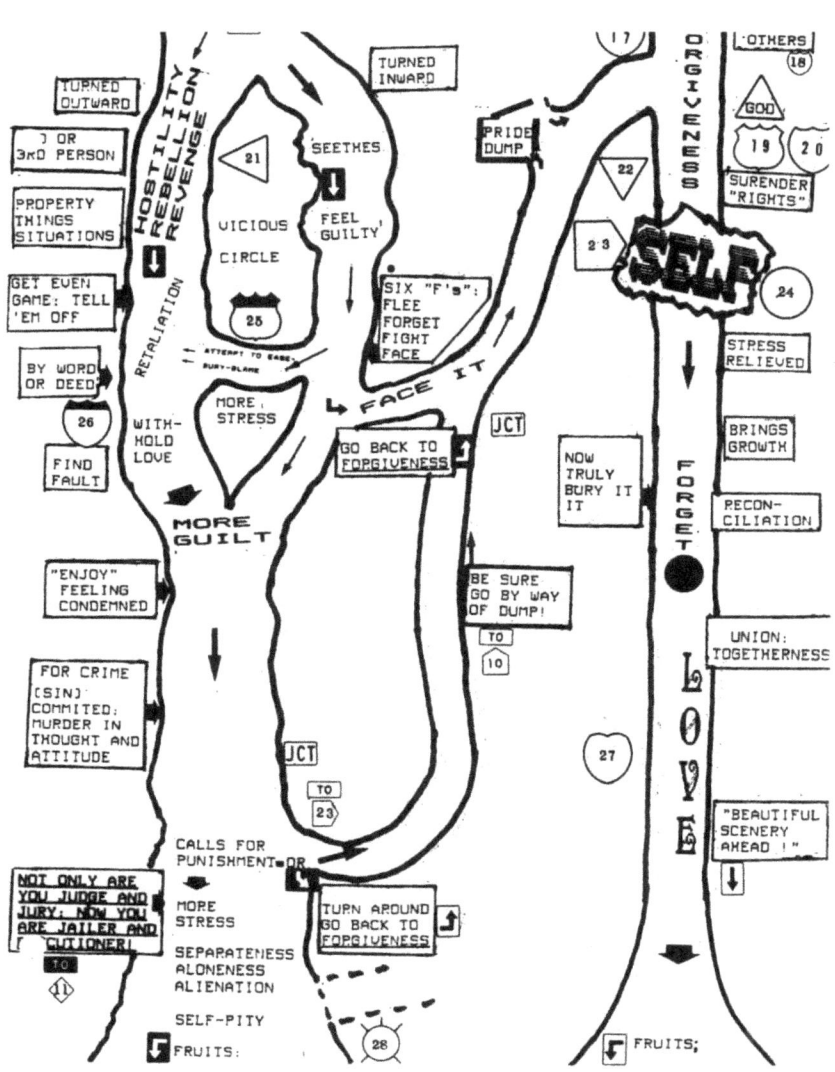

FRUITS; THE HARVEST, (TARES-WEEDS)	FRUITS OF THE GOOD HARVEST

★ MENTAL AND EMOTIONAL

LOST FEELING OF LOVE	LOVING, BELONGINGNESS
POOR OR BAD SELF-IMAGE	GOOD SELF-LOVE
WORRY	A "KNOWING" FEELING
NEGATIVE ATTITUDE	POSITIVE ATTITUDE
SKEPTICISM	SECURITY
TENSION, ANXIETY	RELAXED, SURE
INFERIORITY, SHYNESS	SELF-CONFIDENCE, SELF-RELIANCE
DEPRESSION, LONLINESS	HAPPINESS, COMPANIONSHIP
DESPAIR, DESPONDENCY	OPTIMISTIC, COMPETENT
INDIFFERENCE, DEFEAT	ACTIVE CONCERN FOR SELF AND OTHERS
ANGUISH, PANIC, DIVORCE	GRATIFICATION, TOGETHERNESS
"NERVOUS BREAKDOWN"	CALM, COOL, CONFIDENT
MENTAL SUICIDE (DRUGS)	HIGH, HAPPY AND HEALTHY

★ PHYSICAL

OVERWEIGHT AND HUNGER	TRIM AND FIT AND SATIATED
TIREDNESS	ENERGETIC, INVIGORATED
LOW BACK PAIN	RELIEVED, RELAXED
STOMACH ACHE, ULCER	RESTED, RESTORED
SPASTIC COLON, DIAR.	NORMAL BM, HARDY
HEADACHES, DIZZINESS	COMFORTABLE
INSOMNIA, NERVOUSNESS	SLEEP WELL, SOOTHED NERVES
ALLERGIES, HIVES, ETC	GOOD COUNTENANCE
COLDS, FLU, ETC.	CLEAR HEADED
IMPAIRED VISION	CLEAR VISION
CANCER	REFRESHED, SPIRITED
PRISON	FREEDOM
PHYSICAL SUICIDE (DEATH)	WELLNESS

★ SPIRITUAL

IMPAIRED **TRIUMVIRATE**	
LOVE, ROMANCE, SEX	LOVE, GIVING
REJECTED	ACCEPTANCE, HARMONY
FEAR	FAITH, HOPE
SCORN	FORGIVING, CARING
SHAME, SELF-CONTEMPT	SELF-RESPECT, DIGNITY
CYNICAL, SARCASTIC	APPRECIATION, GRATITUDE
SPITEFUL, CRITICAL	SHARING, ACTIVE CONCERN
HATE, HOSTILITY	SENSE OF ACHIEVEMENT
JEALOUSY	TRUSTING, WORTHINESS
MORE GUILT, (VICIOUS CIRCLE)	FREEDOM, PEACE, CONTENTMENT, JOY
IMPAIRED STATE OF BEING	STATE OF WELL-BEING
SPIRITUAL SUICIDE	RESPONSIBLE, SUCCESS
(SENSUALITY, OCCULT, ETC.)	HAPPY, ABUNDANT LIFE

HURT MAP   LAF BOOK

"ROAD SIGNS" References

(1) "--Choose this day whom you will serve."Joshua 24:15. Refer to "Map To Victory-", page 16 & 17 of LAF BOOK. Also see Norman Wright's "Steps For Handling Frustration or Anger",page 51 "An Answer To Anger And Frustration". Be sure to write the answers that come to your mind. Don Polston in "There Can Be A New You" gives us six steps for overcoming depression and anger:

    "(1) Don't take life so seriously.
    (2) Remember, what you truly need you'll get.
    (3) Keep in mind that if you are angry, someone is
         controlling your life.
    (4) Anger is saying, 'You're my equal.' Whomever you are angry with
         is on your level.
    (5) Ask the question, 'What would Jesus do?'
    (6) Allow the Holy Spirit to control you by
         surrendering and praying."

(2) FRUSTRATION and ANGER: TWINS. "Lord give me the wisdom to know the difference". (St. Francis)

(3) "He who is slow to anger is better than the mighty, and he who rules his spirit than he who takes a city. "Proverbs 16:32.

(4) NO ONE can control you unless you allow it.

(5) Don Polston in "There Can Be A New You" says, "Most people who irritate you or annoy you are ignorant of the good you could be to them. But because they lack understanding, don't fall into the same pit and be like them".

(6) "Hatred stirs up strife, but love covers all offenses".
    Proverbs 10: 12.

(7) "But I say to you that every one who is angry with his brother shall be liable to judgement." Matthew 5:22,"

(8) "Make no friendship with a man given to anger, nor go with a wrathful man, lest you learn his ways and entangle yourself in a snare." Proverbs 22:24&25.

(9) "Forgive and you will be forgiven." Luke 6:37.

(10) "So if you are offering your gift at the altar and there remember that your brother has something against you, leave your gift there before the altar and go; first be reconciled to your brother, and then come offer your gift." Matthew 5: 23&24.

(11) "Judge not, that you be not judged." Matthew 7:1.

(12) "A man of quick temper acts foolishly, but a man of discretion is patient." Proverbs 14:17.

(13) "Set your minds on things that are above, not on things that are on earth." "But now put them all away, anger, wrath, malice, slander and foul talk--". Colossians 3:2,8.

(14) "Let all bitterness and wrath and anger and clamor and slander be put away from you, with all malice, and be kind one to another, tenderhearted, forgiving one another, as God in Christ forgave you." Ephesians 4:31&32.

(15) Again from Don Polston, "All emotional tension can be traced to one of two things: anger or fear." They go hand in hand.

(16) "Refrain from anger, and forsake wrath! Fret not thyself; it tends only to evil." Psalms 37:8.

(17) "Live in harmony with one another;- Repay no one evil for evil, but take thought for what is noble in the sight of all. If possible, so far as depends upon you, live peaceably with all." Romans 12:16-18.

(18) "You have heard that it was said, 'You shall love your neighbor and hate your enemy.' But I say to you, Love your enemies and pray for those who persecute you." Matthew 5:43&44.

(19) "For if you forgive men their trespasses, your heavenly Father also will forgive you." Matthew 6: 14&15.

(20) "If we confess our sins, he is faithful and just, and will forgive our sins and cleanse us from all unrighteousness." I John 1:9.

(21) "Beloved, never avenge yourselves, but leave it to the wrath of God; for it is written, 'Vengeance is mine, I will repay', says the Lord." Romans 12:19

(22) "Do not be overcome by evil, but overcome evil with good." Romans 12:21

(23) John Kanory, Self Image Seminar leader says, "WE are our greatest problem". We need to get "SELF" out of the way!

(24) Don Polston also gives this bit of advice:
   "(1) Truly know who you are.
    (2) Truly seek excellence in your work and character.
    (3) Refuse to accept the blame on the basis of your
         personal worth.
    (4) Consider the source of your blame.
    Maybe they have a problem.

(25) Don Polston, in "There Can Be a New You" states, "The more you blame others, the greater the possibility grows for self-hate. Blaming people usually causes more mistakes which cause more blame". VICIOUS CIRCLE.

(26) RETALIATION BY WORD OR DEED; Can do it four ways: Kill 'em, Blame 'em, Find fault with them,
   Reject completely. (Don't play God.)

(27) "Love is patient and kind; love is not jealous or boastful." I Corinthians 13: 4&5.

(28) When anger reaches this final stage, there is usually no turning around! Forgiveness becomes almost impossible.
   Yet "-- with God nothing will be impossible". Luke 1:37.

WELCOME HOME !

135

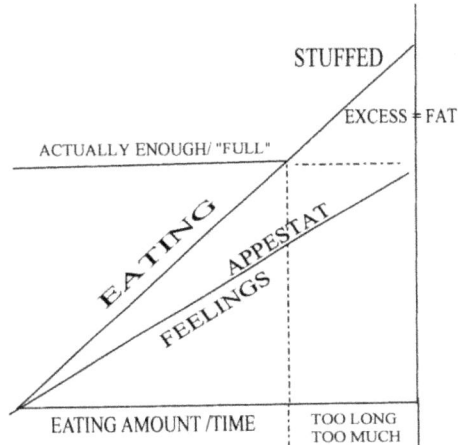

STUFFED

EXCESS = FAT

ACTUALLY ENOUGH/ "FULL"

EATING

APPESTAT

FEELINGS

EATING AMOUNT /TIME

TOO LONG
TOO MUCH

WITH A PICTURE OF THIS CHART IN MIND,
YOU'LL FIND IT EASY AND COMFORTABLE
EATING ONLY ENOUGH AT ANY MEAL TO HOLD
YOU OVER UNTIL THE NEXT MEAL. YOU WILL
NEVER FEEL UNCOMFORTABLE AND STUFFED!

BUT YOU WILL SEE A POSITIVE PERSON
PICTURE AND ~~LAUGH~~ LAUFF FOR JOY AS YOU
LOOK AT YOURSELF IN THE MIRROR!!

Let me now introduce you to the **TOGETHERNESS EXERCISE.** LOVE is TOGETHERNESS.

While sitting, well supported, in a comfortable choir, use your hands to make a pointer with each, index fingers pointing like "pistols."

Bring hands together, forefingers still pointing, but now upward with elbows resting on your chest. Focus attention on the tips of your forefingers. Now count backwards slowly from 7 to 1, RELAX, RELAX, RELAX. Notice as you relax, the tips of your forefingers come together. (At first, you may need to repeat the count to get the best results. As you practice this exercise, you will find yourself relaxing more quickly.) This exercise represents TOGETHERNESS, union, which is brought about by LOVE - a togetherness of inner-mind with outer-mind, subconscious mind with conscious mind, "left brain" with "right brain." Let it represent a union of mind, body and spirit, and union and oneness with the Eternal Love Spirit. As your fingers close, let your eyes close, closing out negative impressions for this moment. You now let this harmony envelop your entire being in a physical, mental and spiritual renewal. Visualize the messages from the mind-brain travelling over the complex nerve communication system to every organ, every muscle, every cell and fiber of your being.

Just a Few moments in this state *of* mind is all that is necessary to reap beautiful benefits. To establish a reasonable length of time, simply count backwards from seventy (70) just as soon as your fingers and eyes close. Your counting should be at about the same rate as your breathing. So just count along with each breath cycle.

(IF you lose count along the way, no problem, just pick up where you think you should be.) When you reach zero in your count down from seventy, immediately count forward to seven. This completes your Togetherness Exercise, emerging you feeling rested, relaxed, refreshed, rejuvenated. You emerge Feeling clear-headed and alert. The count forward to seven is like closing out a program on a computer- your mind-brain-body computer. Always close out to help keep any negatives from being recorded in your computer-memory.

Using this exercise before each session with your LAF CARDS and SCRIPT CARDS makes the affirmations and suggestions even more powerful and effective. You *may* **use** it anytime by itself for your "R and R" **Session** - Relaxation and Rejuvenation. You Find that each time you use it, it becomes more and more effective. As you gain experience, you can shorten the counts and still be very effective.

LAUNCHING YOUR POSITIVE PEP/PIM

HOW TO CREATE and SECURE IN YOUR MIND a desired

POSITIVE PROMPTER/MOTIVATOR – A NEW SCRIPT.
142

HOW TO NEGATE-OVERRIDE AN UNWANTED NEGA-PEP/
NEGA-PIM.

HOW TO GIVE YOURSELF A "TRIGGER" TO LAUNCH YOUR
POSI-PEP/POSI-PIM.

To CREATE and SECURE in your mind a POSITIVE
PROMPTER/MOTIVATOR and make it PREDOMINANT:

First go back to "REWARDS AND BENEFITS" and reread,
or if not completed as yet, NOW is the time definitely do so. Get
the REWARDS and BENEFITS clearly in your mind. The more
EMOTIONAL BENEFITS that you list, the more powerful will be
your POSITIVE PROMPTERS. Read over and over, at least seven
times NOW.

Then think of your "LAF GOAL IMAGE". Pick out what   MEANS
THE MOST TO YOU. Write the complete sentence down. For
example:

"I want to feel attractive."
"I want to look trim and strong."
"I want to have my children and spouse proud of me."
"I want to do more things, to go places.
    These are "Love MESSAGES", ways of expressing love for
yourself, and to those near and dear to you. Notice that they
pertain to your emotions and the mental images of yourself.
These are POSITIVE EMOTIONAL PROMPTERS (PEPs) and
POSITIVE IMAGE MOTIVATORS (PIMs).

Immediately get into a quiet and restful place as you can, and
start the TOGETHERNESS EXERCISE.

143

After counting down seven to one and closing out outside distractions as much as possible, and as you are counting backwards from seventy to one, let your inner mind imagination take you back to a time and place when and where you felt especially good about yourself, to a situation where you felt very happy, especially

self-confident and self-assured, a time when everything was going your way. Picture in your mind your physical well-being, your positive attitude, your step, your voice, and actions. SEE, FEEL and BELIEVE that you are in that same state of mind-brain-body of contentment and happiness. The references to what you've written in the LAF BOOK, what "turns you on", will help bring it more vividly to your mind. NOW WHEN YOU ARE AT THE VERY TOP LEVEL OF THE EXPERIENCE, PHYSICALLY, MENTALLY AND

EMOTIONALLY, take your seven deep breaths, exhaling slowly and saying your cue word-your TRIGGER word. RELAX. At the seventh breath touch the crook of your jaw. (Another unique physical contact may be used to suit you personally. However be sure it is something unusual, something that you would not otherwise normally do). Now go to a similar experience and repeat the process. Then a third. You are tying down and securing the experience as a POSITIVE PREDOMINANT PROMPTER. At the same time you are creating a "TRIGGER" that you can use anytime and anyplace in the future to place yourself back in that powerful positive state of mind. Your physical well-being follows.

144

At times or in situations when you cannot take all seven breaths, by saying your TRIGGER word and/or sound after each breath, along with the touching, you still have an effective TRIGGER. This is a "prompter" to prompt your POSI-PEP/POSI-PIM. IT I S Y O U R " HPNOTIC Q U E ", a signal, a stimulus that incites positive helpful responses and influences your love-self-more behavior. You have the combination of an action (taking the deep breaths), a sound or word and a kinesthetic movement cue. If in the presence of others, it can be done silently and secretly and be Just as effective.

You also have the POWER OF PRE-DECISION, like a posthypnotic suggestion. You are pre-deciding how you will feel and how you will react to certain conditions or in various situations. Then when you are in that condition or situation, you simply carry out the decision that you've already made.

Each time you use this method it will be more effective. You will be experiencing those same high, happy and healthy feelings. This becomes post-hypnotic in effect; like the carrying out of a post-hypnotic suggestion. Repeat this whole exercise at least seven times over a period of a few days.

TO NEGATE A NEGATIVE PROMPTER

Now for some very dramatic experiences. To NEGATE or OVERRIDE an unwanted negative PROMPTER, you simply bring your new POSITIVE PROMPTER and your old negative prompter together! Remembering that the BASIC NEGATIVE PREDOMINANT EMOTIONAL PROMPTER is

145

lack of LOVE or misapplied love, you now do the things to bring about the desired results.

Here again refer back to your LAF NOTE BOOK. Look under "I EAT ", "I EAT WHEN " and "I LOVE ". Review these NEGATIVE PROMPTERS. Write them down also.

Example:

"I eat SWEETS".
"I eat when I'm LONELY". "I eat when I'm ANGRY".
"I LOVE CHOCOLATE".
Now put yourself in one of those situations, or when you find yourself in one of those situations, <u>at the same time</u>, take the seven deep breaths, saying your TRIGGER word and touching the crook of your jaw. It is an instant mood changer. You thus collapse and cancel out the NEGA-PEP/PIM, like letting the air out of a balloon. You are replacing the Nega-PEP/PIM with the Posi-PEP/PIM.

SEVENTY SECONDS (OR LESS)

RELAXATION and REJUVENATION

SESSION

This is also your POS1-PEP and

POS1-PIM TRIGGER.

Inhale and exhale deeply and slowly seven times. Inhale deeply LOVE'S REJUVINATING IMPELLING FORCE, replacing all tension, discord, and other negatives.

As you exhale say your unique special word, "RELAX" and/or make a special sound. Do this after each of the seven breaths. At the end of the seventh breath, touch the crook of your jaw.

FROM: PSALMS 20:4,5 RSV.

MAY HE GRANT YOU YOUR HEART'S DESIRE,

AND FULFILL ALL YOUR PLANS !

MAY WE SHOUT FOR JOY OVER YOUR VICTORY,

AND IN THE NAME OF OUR GOD

SET UP OUR BANNERS!

MAY THE LORD FULFILL ALL YOUR PETITIONS!

In His Name, with LOVE,
Amen
Joe G.. Prescott

www.ingramcontent.com/pod-product-compliance
Lightning Source LLC
Chambersburg PA
CBHW072215290526
45794CB00004B/1755